BRANDED BY LOVE:

A JOURNEY FROM AN OCEAN OF TEARS TO A LIFE OF TRIUMPH

BRANDED BY LOVE:
A JOURNEY FROM AN OCEAN OF TEARS TO A LIFE OF TRIUMPH

PATRICIA SOTO

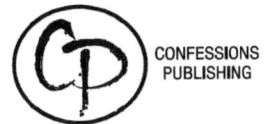

Scripture quotations marked as (AMPC) are taken from the *Holy Bible*: The Amplified Bible, Copyright © 2015 Classic Edition. Publisher: The Lockman Foundation. All Rights Reserved

Scripture quotations marked as (BSB) are taken from the *Holy Bible*, Berean Study Bible BSB, Copyright ©2016, 2018 by Bible Hub Used by Permission. All rights reserved Worldwide.

Scripture quotations marked (CEV) are from the Contemporary English Version, Copyright © 1995 by the American Bible Society. Used by permission.

Scripture quotations marked (CJB) are from the Complete Jewish Bible. Copyright © 1998 by David H. Stern. All rights reserved.

Scripture quotations marked as (CSB) are from the *Holy Bible:* Holman Chrisitain Standard Version. Copyright © 2009 Nashville: Holman Bible Publishers. All rights reserved.

Scripture quotations marked (ESV) are taken from the *Holy Bible*, English Standard Version © 2001 by Crossway Bibles, a division of Good News Publishers. Used by permission. All rights reserved.

Scriptures quotations marked as (EXB) are taken from The Expanded Bible © 2011 by Thomas Nelson Inc. Used by permission. All rights reserved

Scripture quotations marked (GNT) are taken from the *Good News Bible: The Bible in Today's English Version*. © 1976 New York: American Bible Society. All rights reserved.

Scripture quotations marked (KJV) are taken from the *Holy Bible*, King James Version.

Scripture quotations marked (MSG) are taken from the *Holy Bible, The Message Bible* © 2005 Colorado Springs, Co: NavPress.

Scripture quotations marked (NIV) are taken from the *Holy Bible*, New International Version. Zondervan Publishing House © 1984. Used by permission. All rights reserved.

Scripture quotations marked (NKJV) are taken from the *Holy Bible*, New King James Version © 1982 by Thomas Nelson. Used by permission. All rights reserved.

Scripture quotations are taken from the *Holy Bible*, New Living Translation © 2004. Wheaton, III: Tyndale House Publisher.

Scripture quotations marked (TLB) are from The Living Bible. Copyright © 1971. Used by permission of Tyndale House Publisher, Ic., Wheaton, IL 60189. All rights reserved.

Branded By Love: A Journey From An Ocean of Tears To A Life of Triumph

Copyright © Patricia Soto

ISBN: 978-1-7359620-7-8

Printed and bound in the United States of America.

All Rights Reserved. No part of this publication may be reproduced, stored in a retrieval system, or transmitted, in any form or by any means- electronic, mechanical, photocopying, recording, or otherwise- used in any manner whatsoever without the express written permission of the author, Patricia Soto.

Editor: Erick Markley

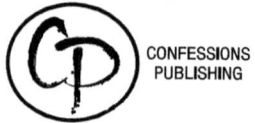

CONFESSIONS PUBLISHING

Confessions Publishing is a subsidiary of Roszien Kay LLC, Lancaster, CA 93536

For information regarding discounts on bulk purchase and all other inquiries, please contact the author directly at authorsoto@gmail.com or godsgardnr42@msn.com

Thank You...

I am grateful beyond words for all that God has done for me and my family my whole life. From tears to a life of abundance, it was only God who could have brought us through. We all would be nowhere, if not for the hand of God. His mercy and goodness know no boundaries. And now we are to be His hands. We are to be His feet. We are to be His voice.

My greatest desire is to do the work of God, whatever that may be in each season of my life. Although I cannot go to all the places where there is a need, I am committed to helping in any way that God leads. In my travels I have witnessed some unbearable living conditions where children are without food, clean water, or clothing. I have seen children living in conditions that break my heart. And I have seen families that will do anything to survive.

At this present time, the Lord has impressed upon me to help ministries that serve on the frontlines—those that bring assistance and the Gospel to families and children in third world countries. These ministries generously provide food, clothing, education and knowledge that improves the living conditions for villages and tribes. For every book purchased, 100% of the proceeds will go to organizations such as: Mother of the Nations, Flood Relief Campaign in Pakistan, African Inland Mission, Mercy Ships, along with any other reputable missionary agency.

Many thanks for purchasing this book and providing hope for a child, a family, and a community...

CONTENTS

PREFACE 1
CHAPTER 1: A TIME FOR EVERYTHING 5
CHAPTER 2: STORMY WEATHER 11
CHAPTER 3: INHERITANCE.. 19
CHAPTER 4: ALL DOWN HILL 23
CHAPTER 5: DEATH AND MERCY 39
CHAPTER 6: BROKEN 49
CHAPTER 7: NEVER-ENDING 59
CHAPTER 8: REBELLION'S END 73
CHAPTER 9: THE RIVER 81
CHAPTER 10: SURRENDERING 89
CHAPTER 11: BEHIND THE SCENES.. 97
CHAPTER 12: I AM BLESSED 111
CHAPTER 13: NOT THIS TIME 121
CHAPTER 14: HIS LOVE 131
CHAPTER 15: HIS LOVE LETTER 151
CHAPTER 16: GOD'S FAITHFULNESS... 171
CHAPTER 17: HIS WORD 185
CHAPTER 18: THE FIRE, THE BATTLEGROUND, THE TESTING ... 199
CHAPTER 19: OBEDIENCE 211
CHAPTER 20: VICTORY 217

CHAPTER 21: OUR JOB	233
CHAPTER 22: MY ROCK	237
CHAPTER 23: RESTORATION	243
CHAPTER 24: SEASON OF PLUNDER	247
EPILOGUE	257
ACKNOWLEDGMENT	265
ABOUT THE AUTHOR	267

PREFACE

Out of obedience to God and a desire to please Him, I started this book on January 1st, 2020. I really just wanted to record my story because I love to write, but it turned out to be so much more. God wanted this to be an intimate time between us for Him to minister His love for me and that is exactly what He did every moment of this process.

In every word, on every page I poured out my heart in worship to God sharing with you things that I have never said out loud. I really never expected to publish this book or ever have anybody read it because it was so personal, between me and God. But God was adamant about healing me completely so all of it had to be exposed; all of it had to come to His light. I thought this would be a painful process, but it was not. This was an amazing journey that God took me through and after writing this book I realized I could never have kept it to myself.

Many hours of healing and restoration happened during this time. Many hours of prayer and tears went into this book. I had to take you to the depths of the valley of the shadow of death that I walked through for 20y ears, in order to show you the greatness of God's glory! It was 20 years of torment.

It was 20 years of tears. It was 20 years of heartache. It was 20 years of living in fear. But every step I took during the 20 year period was important to what God needed to teach me.

This book was written without me taking one writer's class, any instruction, or any help from anyone. So please forgive me for any roughness in the writing. It had to be God alone that spoke to me and through me. His voice was my only leading.

The process of writing this book was one in which I am familiar with. It's the same process He took me through with photography. With photography, I have shot so many different events and I have shot in different countries on missionary trips, but have never had any formal training. To be very honest with you, my brain cannot retain the complex or even basic training of photography, so relying on knowledge is impossible. I must rely on God's voice for everything.

Photography was one of my training grounds that God taught me to obey His voice, even while I was still walking in disobedience. This was preparation for when He had to lead me into battles relying only on Him. It has been God alone that has taught me and has led me every step of the way.

With writing this book, just like with photography, God led me every step of the way. In fact the steps and the answers were there for years written in my journals. But each piece did not make sense until the Holy Spirit put it all together to form one complete picture.

PREFACE

All it took was obedience to His voice. I didn't even realize I was already walking it all out, until I started writing this book. His light now shines on every path I take.

October 1st, 2020 which is a significant anniversary for me; It is the date I finished writing this book. This specific date had been for years, a struggle of hope and fear because it was the day I was first diagnosed with breast cancer. It is also the beginning of the annual "Breast Cancer Awareness" month so there are reminders everywhere I go, every year. Now exactly 12 years later I am releasing to the atmosphere my victory from this day.

Because my mother died 10 years after the first time she was diagnosed with breast cancer, passing this milestone was huge. Statistics say you will not live 10 years after a cancer diagnosis. For so long the devil used the 10 year mark as my expiration date to bring fear and mental torment. He harassed me day in and day out. But God turned it completely around to a day of freedom and joy for my life! This victory at this time was crucial for my life and for my daughter's and granddaughter's lives because breast cancer has been defeated in my lineage forever.

It may seem like one small victory to some, but it was enormous in the scope of things for me. It ended an era in my life that only God could have brought me through. And because of this whole shift in my spirit, it has caused me many more victories after this book was finished. This victory has led me down a path of continuous victories in everything I face.

As I am sitting here writing this preface, I am reflecting on the past 20 years of battles I went through. I had thought for so long it was a waste of my life and years of torture for no reason, and yet *every moment HE WAS FAITHFUL*. Suddenly God speaks to my heart, "Now 20 years of blessings!" What an amazing Father! What a faithful God! What a beautiful Lord!

I cannot say it enough, seeking God will bring you so much more joy and satisfaction than anything and everything in this world! Nothing compares to Him! Nothing compares to His presence! Nothing will ever affect you as the sweetness of His voice! Nothing compares to being fully surrendered! Nothing compares to losing your life!

Please take the time to read each scripture and allow God to speak to you. There were hundreds of scripture I wanted to add to this book and I could go on forever about how wonderful God is and the great things He has done, but it is your story that must be told now. It is your own battle you must have victory in. It is the hidden treasures in the Word of God that you must find on your own now. It is your path that you must pursue. And it is His voice you must follow . . .

CHAPTER 1:
A TIME FOR EVERYTHING

"There is a time for everything, and a season for every activity under the heavens: a time to be born and a time to die, a time to plant and a time to uproot, a time to kill and a time to heal, a time to tear down and a time to build, a time to weep and a time to laugh, a time to mourn and a time to dance, a time to scatter stones and a time to gather them, a time to embrace and a time to refrain from embracing, a time to search and a time to give up, a time to keep and a time to throw away, a time to tear and a time to mend, a time to be silent and a time to speak, a time to love and a time to hate, a time for war and a time for peace."

(Ecclesiastes 3:1-8 NIV)

All throughout our lives, things around us are transforming. Our personal lives never stay the same and most people usually adapt well. Most changes or seasons in our lives come on slowly and almost all transitions are smooth. Sometimes, we don't even realize we are in a new season until we have been in it for quite some time.

Not my life—ever! Sometimes, I sensed new seasons coming, and sometimes, I was oblivious. Sometimes, I heeded the warnings, and other times, I just ignored what God was trying to prepare me for. Either way, it was always like a giant wave hitting me, knocking me over, gasping for air. Many times, it was so exhilarating, but quite often it was so devastating, like a kick in the head that I did not see coming.

After leaving a very short and bad marriage to a violent man, I had met and married at church at the age of 21, I wanted nothing to do with people, especially men. So, I just threw myself on the altar of God, literally dedicating my life to serving him. Feelings of worthlessness and loneliness overwhelmed me and had to be destroyed, and I wanted that past year of my life to be erased from my memory. All I longed for was to get lost in God. He had already done so much for me and my baby daughter, like keeping us alive and safe through some horrible times. So, I knew there was nowhere else to turn. I had a deep sense that I now belonged to him and him alone, which was fine with me!

God led me to a tiny white church on a corner in a little town that I had seen for years, but never paid attention to. Once on the inside of this little building, it seemed so big. It was a giant inside. Everything about it, including the faith and love of these people, were larger than life. I walked in not knowing what to expect and was so surprised at the presence of God there. It was powerful, unlike anything I had ever encountered. I knew my life would change forever from that moment on. So, I settled myself in quite easily.

There, I served in ministry, rededicated my heart, learned so much about the power of God, got delivered of all the past, and made many new friends. I fit in and was accepted so easily, like I had always been there, like I was family. The anointing of God was incredible. The love of God was prevalent. The worship swept me away deeper and deeper, always leaving me wanting more. I couldn't get enough of God's Spirit. Putting down roots and building relationships was easy because I thought I would be there forever, but I was wrong. Less than a year later, suddenly, I felt a change was coming soon. As a result, I became restless trying to wait patiently to see what God was going to do next and yet expecting the worst.

Changes came in a moment's notice. I was not looking for a relationship because I was so content with my life for the first time ever. I felt alive and in love with God and I wanted nothing to change, but God had other plans. Suddenly, I was in a whirlwind relationship; I met a man and fell in love, literally within days. Mario was living with his mom when we met, going to school, driving a little blue station wagon, making very little money, and he had a small child. These were red flags for most women in those days and for my friends and parents too, who were very blatant with their concerns. But thank God, He sees beyond who we are now.

God was wasting no time, and neither was Mario. Still a little apprehensive, I just trusted God knew what He was doing and let God work in us. We married only six months later in a small chapel on a beautiful fall day, bringing two little families together so fast my head was spinning. Mario had a sweet 5-year-old daughter, and I had a beautiful 4-year-old daughter, both of which had lost their other parent.

Soon after, we had two more children, we were working at good jobs, making great money, enjoying nice homes and cars, and had a very active life. Our days were filled with birthday parties and Disneyland trips, minivans and beach days, camping and church activities, dog shows and drive-ins, loads of never-ending laundry and carts overflowing with groceries. I was so happy. We had my family close by and things couldn't have been any better.

My dad and Mario became garage sailing buddies, always gone for hours every Saturday morning, bringing home ridiculous junk every time. We gave freely, served at church faithfully, and were enjoying the abundance God had blessed us with. Our kids ran around the neighborhood enjoying so many friends from different cultures and religions and were always involved in activities. Life was beautiful. Favor and blessings surrounded us everywhere we went, and we were never ungrateful. We knew all we had was because of God!

Over the first 12 years, the seasonal changes in our lives were very sudden, but fun for all of us. Jobs changed suddenly, and with it, new cities, new friends, new churches, and new schools. Sometimes, when we moved because of work to a new area, I would grab all the kids, the dogs, and a bunch of snacks, and would drive around until we picked a new neighborhood we all liked to live in, not knowing anything about it or anyone. My kids did well with every change, and we just made the best of every situation. It was exciting, and I always looked forward to the next big adventure in our lives. Everything was perfect.

Meditation Scriptures

Isaiah 41:10 BSB

I brought you from the ends of the earth and called you from its farthest corners. I said, 'You are My servant.' I have chosen and not rejected you. Do not fear, for I am with you; do not be afraid, for I am your God. I will strengthen you; I will surely help you; I will uphold you with My right hand of righteousness. Behold, all who rage against you will be ashamed and disgraced; those who contend with you will be reduced to nothing and will perish. You will seek them but will not find them. Those who wage war against you will come to nothing. For I am the LORD your God, who takes hold of your right hand and tells you: Do not fear, I will help you.

Psalms 40:5 BSB

Many, O LORD my God, are the wonders You have done, and the plans You have for us— none can compare to You— if I proclaim and declare them, they are more than I can count.

Jeremiah 29:11

For I know the plans I have for you,' declares the Lord, 'plans to prosper you and not to harm you, plans to give you hope and a future.

James 1:17

Every good and perfect gift is from above, coming down from the Father of the heavenly lights, who does not change like shifting shadows.

Matthew 6:33 NLT

Seek the Kingdom of God above all else, and live righteously, and he will give you everything you need.

Psalm 92:12-15 NLT

But the godly will flourish like palm trees and grow strong like the cedars of Lebanon. For they are transplanted to the Lord's own house. They flourish in the courts of our God. Even in old age they will still produce fruit; they will remain vital and green. They will declare, "The Lord is just!

He is my rock! There is no evil in him!"

Psalms 16:11 NLT

You will show me the way of life, granting me the joy of your presence and the pleasures of living with you forever.

CHAPTER 2:
STORMY WEATHER

"My soul is in the midst of lions; I lie down amid fiery beasts—the children of man, whose teeth are spears and arrows, whose tongues are sharp swords. Be exalted, O God, above the heavens! Let your glory be over all the earth! They set a net for my steps; my soul was bowed down. They dug a pit in my way, but they have fallen into it themselves."

(Psalm 57:4-6 ESV)

Unaware of the shift in the atmosphere, and totally unprepared, lightning struck out of nowhere. Maybe there were warnings, but I was not paying attention. Just like in any paradise, the storms do come swiftly, the hurricane season can be relentless, changing everything you have ever known, leaving the landscape of your life unrecognizable. You can get hit on every side and wonder if you are still standing or even breathing.

For me, this season came instantaneously. One day, life was beautiful, and the very next moment, I was being swept away by a flash flood, struggling to stay alive and drowning fast. I couldn't grasp on to anything to save me, not even God. This was just the beginning of a long season. This storm, this darkness, this horrible valley of death, began in 1999. It wasn't until many years later that I realized that I had walked around blind, surrounded by death's darkness for 20 years.

I was working at a very large local medical group, enjoying a great job in the finance department. This job came with status, authority, money, and many good friends. I only worked till 2:30 because I worked faster and more accurately than most people, and as the favorite assistant to the director of finance, I could make my own hours. After having a great day, I stood up to leave, when a shooting pain went from my chest to my abdomen to my leg, on the right side of my body. It was so intense I could not bear it. Screaming in pain, I almost passed out as I buckled over.

A young man that worked in the office next to me began to panic and then ran off to go get my friend and my boss, leaving me all alone in agony. I couldn't move or walk or even talk. All I remember was terrible fear and excruciating pain. I had no idea what this was or why this was happening to me.

For the most part, I was healthy and pretty active. Crying in pain, I was now being rolled out of the office down a long corridor in my office chair to my friend Doreen's car. I couldn't move without the pain intensifying, but somehow, I got in the car and we took off to the emergency room.

Hours of tests and more tests, and exams of every opening of my body, revealed I was pregnant, but I knew I couldn't be. Something was terribly wrong. My husband arrived in shock, and we were both astonished at the news. I already had 4 kids and had had my tubes cut and tied ten years before, right after my son was born. They said, "congratulations," while I lay there crying in pain. The doctor diagnosed me with cramps and said to go home and call my OB/GYN doctor in the morning, but I was getting worse.

Before I could get up to leave, the unthinkable happened. Soon, I knew I was dying, and I lost all control of my bladder and bowels. I was going into shock. Shivering so bad and so humiliated, I think I was yelling at my husband to get out of the room, I could not believe he was seeing me this way, but I don't know if that really happened or not. I was going out of my mind with the horrible pain and trying to stay conscious. All I could say was "Jesus." Slowly, my body calmed down, and after the nurse cleaned me up, they sent me home.

Later that night, laying crumpled up in bed, still in pain, I was crying out to God, begging him for mercy. Somehow, some way, I survived the night of excruciating torment, barely able to move. Was God hearing me? I thought I had walked with him for many years, but my faith was now out of desperation only, and not out of relationship, preparation, or revelation any longer—I now had nowhere else to turn to. I realized how far I had wandered off course and how shaky my foundation was. The busyness of life had pushed God to the back burner. Praying and reading the Word had become a pastime done occasionally, and the relationship between me and God was on a "as needed" basis. In that moment, I needed him. I had no idea why this happened, but I believed I was at fault somehow.

I returned to the doctors. Once there, they rushed me into surgery early the next day. My doctor found I had a tubal pregnancy that had ruptured, and I was bleeding internally since the day before. This should have killed me by now. The ER should have never sent me home. I cried because I knew that it was a baby boy inside of me, but that neither of us could survive this ordeal if I held on to him. As I lay there shaking, silent tears running down my face, I named him Isaiah, "Yahweh is salvation."

It was a miracle he was even conceived. The thought of him shattered my heart. Deep inside of me, his little heart was beating, and his little hands were reaching out, but he would soon die. This was too much for my heart to handle. His little face I would never kiss. I wanted him to live more than I wanted me to live. I wanted to hold him. I wanted to see his little smile, but I knew I never would.

When I woke that evening, my abdomen was cut from one side to the other, from hip bone to hip bone. Giant staples were all the way across my stomach. I was in so much pain that I could not cry. Medication did nothing for me, this pain was beyond physical. It radiated from my broken heart to my whole body. My baby was gone, but I was alive. A precious love was ripped out of my heart before it could be given to the little person it was meant for. I was in anguish for my baby boy that I desperately longed for.

I grieved for my little Isaiah that I would never know. Mourning, healing, and dealing with intense guilt at the same time was not easy. It took me so long to heal physically, but the emotional trauma lasted so much longer. I buried it deep within my unrepairable heart.

After my surgery, I tried to move on with my life, thinking I was past what happened and was healthy again. But the trauma and grief ate away at me for years. Minor physical problems began to pop up regularly, but I kept going. We had four kids, and a few extra, living with us at any given time. I always came home from work to neighborhood kids all over our house, eating out of my fridge, jumping all over my furniture, swimming in my pool, and sleeping on my floor with my big lazy Rottweiler, Nico. I loved it, even though I still yearned for my baby that would never know this wonderful life. There was still so much pain in my heart when I would think about him or even see the huge ugly scar on my abdomen.

Meditation Scriptures

Psalm 59:3a NLT

They have set an ambush for me. fierce enemies are out there waiting, Lord.

Psalm 69:29-30 NLT

I am suffering and in pain. Rescue me, O God, by your saving power. Then I will praise God's name with singing, and I will honor him with thanksgiving.

Proverbs 10:25

When the storms of life come, the wicked are whirled away, but the godly have a lasting foundation.

Psalm 23 NLT

The Lord is my shepherd; I have all that I need. He lets me rest in green meadows; he leads me beside peaceful streams. He renews my strength. He guides me along right paths, bringing honor to his name. Even when I walk through the darkest valley, I will not be afraid, for you are close beside me. Your rod and your staff protect and comfort me. You prepare a feast for me in the presence of my enemies. You honor me by anointing my head with oil. My cup overflows with blessings. Surely your goodness and unfailing love will pursue me all the days of my life, and I will live in the house of the Lord forever.

STORMY WEATHER

Psalms 34:18 YLT

Near is Jehovah to the broken of heart, And the bruised of spirit He saveth.

CHAPTER 3:
INHERITANCE

"In him we have obtained an inheritance, having been predestined according to the purpose of him who works all things according to the counsel of his will, so that we who were the first to hope in Christ might be to the praise of his glory."

(Ephesians 1:11-12 ESV)

This all came suddenly, just a few months after burying my mom while I was still mourning her and dealing with so much guilt. She had had breast cancer twice and lived only 10 years after her first diagnosis. I knew my own fate was sealed after this, but figured it would be in my 70's like her. This was the inheritance I believed she left me and that I would leave to my daughters. This was where my faith was at, and the time when the door opened for the enemy to come in. This demon followed me everywhere, harassing me for years. My mom had endured a lifetime of physical and mental battles and family trauma, including tragic deaths, murder, incest, rape, abuse, and many relatives born out of incest. But she was a strong woman that never cried or agonized over what she went through, so I thought.

She had a son from a previous marriage that was taken away by the father, which I know broke her completely. She never talked about any of it or anything that might cause her pain. The walls she built were sky high to protect herself from getting hurt again. She held on to unforgiveness until the day she got saved, just hours before she died. Mom had been so shattered that she could not let anyone too close. Her fortress built out of pain and torment kept her safe, but she herself did not know the way out, and it imprisoned her heart and soul for decades.

When I was caring for her when she was in hospice, I had no real understanding of what she was going through or what she had gone through with so many surgeries, radiation, and chemo. She experienced so much nausea, severe burn marks on her chest, loss of hair, exhaustion, and pain, and I believed I was looking at my future in her. I remember when I was a child, she had been laid up in bed on her stomach for months after 7 spinal surgeries. I didn't know the depths of her misery or understand how sad she must have felt now knowing she was dying and having to leave behind all her grandbabies. Numbly, I just focused on the duties I had to do; although my heart was breaking, I could not tell her that.

Affection was not something we showed in our family, nor did we express our emotions. We were fiercely loyal, faithful, and generous, but there was very little warmth behind it. I didn't realize that with physical battles, the relentless heavy mental battles that accompany sickness and disease is just as hard, if not harder and last so much longer than the disease at times. My mom was the toughest person I knew. I assumed she was fine even though she didn't know God. Never did I consider her deeper feelings and pain during this time.

I was not there for her when she needed me most. Caring for her was done out of love, but we both barely spoke of our emotions. This in itself is a tragedy. It is my biggest regret and caused me so much guilt for years. Thankfully, she received Jesus shortly before her death. Years of bitterness and pain lifted from her shoulders, and you could see the transformation instantly. Now knowing where she was going, she would call out to God from her hospital bed, for Him to hurry up and come get her. She wanted to be out of pain physically and I wanted that for her too.

Meditation Scriptures

2 Corinthians 1:3-4 BSB

Blessed be the God and Father of our Lord Jesus Christ, the Father of compassion and the God of all comfort, who comforts us in all our troubles, so that we can comfort those in any trouble with the comfort we ourselves have received from God.

Micah 7:18 NLT

Where is another God like you, who pardons the guilt of the remnant, overlooking the sins of his special people? You will not stay angry with your people forever, because you delight in showing unfailing love. Once again you will have compassion on us. You will trample our sins under your feet and throw them into the depths of the ocean!

CHAPTER 4:
ALL DOWN HILL

"And everyone who hears these words of Mine and does not do them, will be like a foolish (stupid) man who built his house on the sand. And the rain fell, and the floods and torrents came, and the winds blew and slammed against that house; and it fell—and great and complete was its fall."

(Matthew 7:26-27 AMP)

We were still active in our church: hosting church parties, giving out lots of food to the hungry, helping in the kids ministries and just believing that we were committed to living a godly life. I really didn't give much thought to whether I was walking in God's will or how my relationship with Him was. Everything seemed to be superficial, including my friends; I had no real relationships with anybody at church. It all seemed to be satisfactory with no desire to go further any longer. Surrounded by a cloud of oppression, I went on with my life. When I look back now, it was as though God was my neighbor, saying, "Hi, how are you?" in passing and occasionally chatting trying not to get too friendly. But when I was in desperate need, I was pounding on his door.

For me, church had become more of a social activity than it was a spiritual need. I was more interested in giving and helping than I was in the Word. My dad had instilled in my DNA the deep desire to give out of a grateful heart and to serve with a strong work ethic and with integrity. I felt that was all I really needed to commit to doing in the kingdom of God. Prayer was what you did at church on Sunday and if you had an urgent need.

It was not always this way for me, but at the churches we went to now, that's all that was taught and required of you. Surrendering your whole life to God was never preached. Living holy was something only the preacher did. Although we didn't live like the world, my heart was not fully committed to God. Never satisfied, we went from church to church, never really setting down deep roots, never really growing. At least, I didn't. I did want a family where I could be planted, accepted, and grow, but that really never happened. Always feeling like an outsider, I lost interest in almost everything to do with God.

One day in worship, I was standing there wondering why I was worshiping, why I was serving day in and day out and nothing ever changed. No one ever changed. No one even noticed or cared. No one was getting saved, and this church was not growing spiritually, and we were not reaching out to the community. I felt more than stagnate, I felt dead. I had no friends, no one to talk to, and I felt isolated and alone.

People just wanted to talk about themselves. Everyone hugged and said, "I love you," but no one looked into my eyes. No one acted on that love. I thought that God would not want me to waste my time anymore. Because I had no real connection to anyone, my next decision was easy. I got up and walked out during the middle of service and decided I could live my life with God and not with church or people. I never went back. What a relief I felt when I was free of the burden of others on my life. I would soon find out this was the biggest mistake I ever made. This was the biggest lie from the enemy.

I didn't think it could get worse, but then it got darker. The grief and guilt still tormented me even when I was smiling. Years passed, and I endured so many sudden ongoing physical issues during this time, along with intense mental battles. One right after another, or sometimes all at once. I began to expect it and had faith in disease. It seemed like I was always waiting to see what would go wrong next, the apprehension was killing me.

Each new disease problem came on instantly in full force! One day I had no symptoms, the next day, I would be in terrible pain, or suddenly big lumps would appear out of nowhere. Years of horrible and painful stomach and intestinal problems, gallstone attacks, fibromyalgia, severe sleep apnea, anemia, high blood pressure, many many cancer scares, severe spine and tailbone problems, and deformities, including bulging disc and arthritis in my spine, neck damage from accidents, tendinitis, painful arthritis everywhere, severe muscle cramps in my chest, back and legs, carpal tunnel, frozen joints, nerve damage, pinched nerves, sciatica, painful problems with my feet, torn ligaments, and stabbing pains in my back.

I underwent so many oral surgeries. Along with that, a huge painful tumor on my leg that was making it hard to walk, lumps everywhere, positive pap-smears, ovarian cysts, and many female problems, heart problems that left me almost dead, and many other issues as a result of medications and misdiagnoses.

Adding to all of that, injuries from accidents and multiple falls. I can't even remember what else. I went through test after test, painful procedure after procedure, surgery after surgery. There were many complications from each surgery. I had cameras inside every part of my body, surgical biopsy after biopsy, thousands of needles, and no relief. But so many different diagnoses and a hundred prescriptions. Many of these conditions were incurable and they would tell me you will just have to learn to live with it!

There were a few times when they ripped pieces of my flesh out of my body with no local anesthetic. They put cameras down my throat four times causing me to gag so violently that I kicked the doctor. I endured six grueling colonoscopies. They gave me dyes for scans that made me so sick and dizzy for hours that I could not drive, let alone walk out of the building. I was given injections in my joints that caused more pain than the original problem. It hurt so much to move or think at times. Doctor visits, procedures, tests, surgeries, and ER visits were a constant thing for the next 20 years, and I hated every minute. The agony at times was unreal.

Every time they proclaimed a new diagnosis over me, I accepted it, researched it, and learned to live with it. Believing I was strong because I was surviving all of this, and because I had knowledge. *This knowledge was faith perverted from what God wanted me to believe, it was negative faith, faith in the flesh*. Taking what the devil had proclaimed over me, believing it was now mine, I confessed these death sentences over and over. I can't even remember all the names anymore because there were so many.

Weakly, I would rebuke them and say I was healed in the name of Jesus. I would quote a few scriptures when I was really struggling. People would pray for me time and time again, bottles of oil poured over my head with no change. This long list of diagnoses followed me and choked me like a noose. Every time I said any of the names of these diseases, I felt that noose getting tighter and tighter. No longer could I breath. It was like I could not get out of bed because something new might be wrong with me. I would be in shock when I realized, periodically, that I was not in pain for a short period. With each new confession of destruction over my life, the mental battles intensified until I believed this was all normal for me now.

It wasn't like I was having a symptom and running right away to the doctor for pills. I began to feel like people thought I was making all of this up. These were not diagnoses you could fake. I did not exaggerate the pain or even have a low pain tolerance. There was undeniable evidence of each disease, of the stress, and the pain. I had all my children with very little medication, so I believed I was strong and had a high pain tolerance. Now, these pains were unbearable and unrelenting, and yet I did nothing to stop them.

These diseases either attacked in groups or caused other problems. Sometimes, they were chain reactions. They were storms that came on with force when I least expected it, when I was unprepared. They just suddenly appeared, but I would often wait as long as possible before going to the doctor. There were not many periods in the last 20 years that I was not in constant pain in multiple parts of my body or dealing with several of these issues. Still, I did not take pain pills or any pills for that matter.

Suddenly it got more intense. Out of nowhere, my heart rhythm would increase to well over 220 irregular beats per minute, making me extremely dizzy, exhausted, out of breath, and feeling like my chest was going to explode. Never had I experienced anything like this, or any serious heart problems. The nurse told me I could go into cardiac arrest; sudden death at any moment if they did not get it under control right away.

My heart was so bad, that after they stuck my arm four times trying to get an IV in, they had to stop my heart with medication four times and revive it while I was still awake in order to reset my rhythm. This was HORRIBLE! I was overtaken by the pain and had to keep myself from screaming out and passing out. My body became uncontrollably rigid and twisted and it felt like I was being slowly run over by a truck. The agony was so intense, like death creeping up from my toes inch by inch to my head before they started my heart again with another injection.

This happened at the county jail where I was working and at the Cheesecake Factory in Rancho Cucamonga. When it happened at the Cheesecake Factory, I was so alone, and I was sure I was going to die this time.

When it happened at the jail, I should have been humiliated because I was left bare chested in front of my coworkers (mostly men), while they worked on me and getting ready to shock me if the medications did not work, but I didn't care. I was dying. My little Cuban friend, "Rhino," was such an angel. As soon as I told him over the phone that I didn't feel right, he ran across the whole facility and stayed with me the whole time. He held my hand through it all and tried to keep me covered up.

For the few seconds that my heart was stopped, the world seemed to stand still. I was dead but awake and fully aware of my surroundings. I remember silently screaming inside my head. I didn't see anything spiritual or any white lights or horrible fire—thank God! But I just knew I was dying, and I really didn't care. Anything had to be better than being a slave to paralyzing fear and pain any longer.

These issues were so severe that I could not go back to work for a long time. The rhythms of my heart were so erratic, that a few months after the last incident, I had to have several nerves in my heart cauterized to stop the crazy arrhythmias. Laying on that table wide awake, while I felt the catheter going up inside my artery to my heart, I was so scared that I would die right there while things were such a mess in my life and so scared to live like this anymore. The pain was intense as they were burning away nerves inside of my heart, but the fear was more real than anything. Like a gun was being held to my head, any moment could be my last. I felt so alone and feared that God didn't love me and that was why I was going through all of this.

Over the years, I began to put on weight. It was harder and harder to move as things like spinal deformities, arthritis in my spine, chest, knees and hips, and damage to my neck, legs, and head, slowed me down at times. It made it painful to walk or work out, and yet it was painful to sit still or lay down too long too. Recovery times from all the accidents, surgeries, and procedures would leave me unable to do anything for weeks at a time, and the surgical wounds would hurt for months. A few times, I would have to be rushed to the urgent care for injections because I could not move without screaming when I threw out my back or hips, or when my stomach suddenly revolted.

My heart condition made it hard to do anything strenuous, and many days I could not do anything at all. All the extra weight caused many more horrible things to happen more often. Then the memories of my mom suffering through years of spinal surgery would haunt me. Arthritis, swelling, muscle spasms, nerve pain, and torn tendons in my feet just added to my reasons to not try to lose the weight.

Every time I looked in the mirror I was so disgusted with myself that I stopped looking. I hated everything I saw: my face, my hair (now very grey), all my scars, my body. I stopped making excuses and stopped trying. The more weight I gained, the harder it was to move, so I gained even more. This cycle was only made worse with each new disease. No, I did not eat a lot! No, I am not lazy. Although I have a sweet tooth, I do not binge eat. A kid's meal at any restaurant was very filling to me, and I could never finish an adult sized meal. After years of constant fasting when I first got saved, my stomach had shrunk to that of a 5-year-old. My 7-year-old granddaughter ate more than me. There was no sense in me going to a buffet because I could only eat very little food.

With my hormones, and possibly my thyroid out of balance, the inevitable happened. The inability to be active at times made me so frustrated. And yes, I did try to lose weight, but nothing happened. The scar tissue all over my body limited me in stretching and exercise, so I gave up. I just figured I was destined to be fat, sick, and ugly.

The depression and anxiety I experienced as a result of everything was never-ending. They devoured my life, and nothing brought any relief. It was like I was drowning slowly over and over again, dying from uncontrollable emotions.

At the same time, I was crippled with fear. Fear that was so real: fear of living like this for years, fear of death, fear of pain, fear of more procedures, fear of every disease, fear of doctors, fear of being alone. This consuming fear was not of the unknown, but fear of what I knew was possible and what was probable, what I saw happen in my mother's life from the time I was small till the day she died.

This affected every area of my life, especially my marriage. I always thought of myself as a strong person. Oftentimes, I believed I was handling all of this very well, but in reality, I was not facing it, and this was radiating to others in my life. I had nobody, and I mean nobody, that I could talk to for so many years. Who could understand my heart? Who would even listen? The more I needed to talk, the more I pushed my husband away. How could he ever understand any of what I had endured to this point when he had always been healthy and mentally stable.

My husband was getting more and more distant, or maybe it was me. On the outside, we looked like we were living a blessed life. But on the inside, the battles raged continuously. We fought a lot, and I never held back my words. His solution was to just ignore me and go to bed, or quote lots of scripture to me, which fueled my anger and resentment even more. Kind words or even compassion when I was going through things was a thing of the past. It was as though all that I was enduring was trivial to him. Anytime he reached out to me, I pushed him away. I couldn't stand him around me, but I needed his affection so badly.

He believed that if he took care of my physical needs, like food, helping me with the house, etc., that that was a lot and that that was enough. But nothing was enough. It would not have mattered what he did or didn't do because there was no way to understand what I needed. I didn't know what I needed. There was no way for him to take care of me. I had no idea what I wanted. This was way too much for me and for him, and it only got worse.

The fear, loneliness, and the growing hatred in my heart was consuming me in every way. It burned through my mind and made me bitter and angry all the time. Although not at God, but at my life, at my body and my husband. There was no more laughter, no more swimming parties, no more kids everywhere. There were no more family meals or family parties. The silence was torture, and the emptiness was so agonizing.

As my kids began to leave home and go off to college, they seemed to be good through all of this, but none of them were walking with God. This was not really a concern for me at the time. I wanted them to serve God, but I was dealing with too many other things to think about them. As long as they were alive and healthy, I had no energy to be concerned about them. I was too focused on myself.

That is what the devil wanted along with my own life. You see, when I walked out of that church, I was in the exact position the devil wanted me in, but not only for me. Being out of the perfect will of God is a dangerous place. Now my children and my marriage as well as my health were in his reach because we were no longer united. He could mess with my whole life and everyone in it. I gave him an open door to my children and every generation after that. So, he took what he could from my family during this time. Everything I did, gave the devil more authority over my life.

I still had a sense that God was still with me, but not close; it was like He was watching to see what I was going to do next from a distance. He could intervene, but I really didn't believe He would do that for me because I was not walking with Him. Although I still talked to God, I wondered if He heard me at all. I never questioned God about why I was going through this because I had already seen so many good people go through some horrible things, including my mom. I figured we were all destined to suffer for no reason. Prayers were that of desperate pleas to take it all away. I had no knowledge of what God had really promised me and who He really was. I didn't know God at all or His heart.

Meditation Scriptures

Proverbs 22:9 BSB

A generous man will be blessed, for he shares his food with the poor

Psalm 92:12-13 NLT

But the godly will flourish like palm trees
and grow strong like the cedars of Lebanon.
For they are transplanted to the Lord's own house.
They flourish in the courts of our God.

Nehemiah 9:17 NASB

They refused to listen, And did not remember Your wondrous deeds which You had performed among them; So they became stubborn and appointed a leader to return to their slavery in Egypt But You are a God of forgiveness, Gracious and compassionate, Slow to anger and abounding in lovingkindness; And You did not forsake them.

Romans 7:24 HB

What a wretched man I am! Who will rescue me from this dying body?

Proverbs 24:11 HB

Rescue those being taken off to death,
and save those stumbling toward slaughter.

Luke 13:11 NHEB

And look, a woman who had a spirit of infirmity eighteen years, and she was bent over, and could in no way straighten herself up.

Psalm 18:4-5 MSG

The hangman's noose was tight at my throat;
devil waters rushed over me.
Hell's ropes cinched me tight;
death traps barred every exit.

Ezekiel 36:25-27 NLT

"Then I will sprinkle clean water on you, and you will be clean. Your filth will be washed away, and you will no longer worship idols. And I will give you a new heart, and I will put a new spirit in you. I will take out your stony, stubborn heart and give you a tender, responsive heart. And I will put my Spirit in you so that you will follow my decrees and be careful to obey my regulations.

Psalms 27:19 NKJV

As in water face reflects face,
So a man's heart reveals the man.

Isaiah 30:18 AMP

Therefore the Lord waits [expectantly] and longs to be gracious to you,
And therefore He waits on high to have compassion on you.

For the Lord is a God of justice;
Blessed (happy, fortunate) are all those who long for Him [since He will never fail them]

Psalms 49:15 NLT

But as for me, God will redeem my life. He will snatch me from the power of the grave.

Psalm 43:5

Why are you in despair, my soul? Why are you disturbed within me? Hope in God, because I will praise him once again, since his presence saves me and he is my God.

Isaiah 49:15-16

Can a mother forget the baby at her breast and have no compassion on the child she has borne? Though she may forget, I will not forget you! See, I have engraved you on the palms of my hands; your walls are ever before me.

Job 30:27 ESV

My inward parts are in turmoil and never still;
days of affliction come to meet me.

Isaiah 46:4 BSB

Even to your old age, I will be the same, and I will bear you up when you turn gray. I have made you, and I will carry you; I will sustain you and deliver you.

Psalms 27:13 NKJV

I would have lost heart, unless I had believed That I would see the goodness of the LORD In the land of the living.

Zechariah 9:12 NLT

Come back to the place of safety, all you prisoners who still have hope! I promise this very day that I will repay two blessings for each of your troubles.

Ephesians 4:26:27

When angry, do not sin; do not ever let your wrath (your exasperation, your fury or indignation) last until the sun goes down. Leave no [such] room or foothold for the devil [give no opportunity to him].

Exodus 34:6-7 NLT

The LORD passed in front of Moses, calling out, "Yahweh! The LORD! The God of compassion and mercy! I am slow to anger and filled with unfailing love and faithfulness. I lavish unfailing love to a thousand generations.

I forgive iniquity, rebellion, and sin. But I do not excuse the guilty. I lay the sins of the parents upon their children and grandchildren; the entire family is affected— even children in the third and fourth generations."

CHAPTER 5:
DEATH AND MERCY

"Those who live according to the flesh set their minds on the things of the flesh; but those who live according to the Spirit set their minds on the things of the Spirit. The mind of the flesh is death, but the mind of the Spirit is life and peace."

(Romans 8:5-6 BSB)

One day, I noticed that my lack of caring anymore and my fear were disappearing. What I thought was strength was quickly growing within me. Little by little, I was able to endure more and more with no fear. My heart was so callous, which I thought was great because things no longer affected me emotionally. Step by step, I was becoming indifferent to it all. This was not God I later realized, but the enemy. It was not strength, but I was entering into a living comatose state. I was now building my own fortress just like my mother's, where nothing from this world could affect me anymore. The things that tormented me were now my only friends.

Giving up and surrendering to death was the only thing that brought me relief. I welcomed it, and it gave me a very false sense of peace when all it was was lost hope. This distorted peace was spiritual death. Death was something I was looking forward to, and I often envisioned it. Death was my only way out, and I put all my faith in that.

The devil was circling me, throwing at me anything he could to take me out. I knew he wanted me dead, and I really didn't see a problem with that. It never crossed my mind why he was trying to kill me. I figured I would go to heaven because I had gotten saved so long ago and knew of God, so I wasn't worried. My husband would probably be glad he was off the hook if I died and not having to care for me or even look at me. There were many single women in the church that would jump at the chance to marry him because he offered security in his job and a home which many did not have. My husband could have walked out, and I would have been unable to stop him or fight for him. I wasn't going to stop death or fight it.

When cars came at me on the road and accidents were imminent, I didn't try to move. I figured death would be instant. I had so many near misses while driving; it was almost like the devil was teasing me with instant death and relief from this torment. When I crossed the street, I never looked both ways, or even waited for the lights to change. This all felt normal to me now. I had given up on myself and my life, but God had not.

Once death infiltrated my mind, there was no limit to it. Little by little, I was dying. I had thoughts of suicide as well and homicide every day. The possibility of someone dying close to me was not disturbing to me. Graphic images of horrible accidents plagued my mind every time I drove down the road. I had constant evil thoughts of how I would kill somebody on the street and be able to get away with it. Photos or documentaries of death and any murder movies intrigued me, and I was not surprised when anything went wrong anymore.

So what if I had another disease. I just did not care. The visions of my funeral were commonplace. I even looked into physician assisted suicide and the laws. Things were so very wrong in my life, in my mind, and in my heart. Everything did not turn out how it was supposed to.

Then out of nowhere, God in his great mercy, sent me a wonderful blessing, my first grandson, Eli! I was so happy. I figured my life had suddenly changed. Now it would turn around, and I could live again. When he was born, I could not let go of him. His grandpa wanted to hold him, but letting go of him was like letting go of everything good in my life, even if it was just for a few minutes. I could not let go of the hope and the real peace he brought me. Seeing his little smile overwhelmed me with so much joy. Every chance I got, he was by my side and in my arms.

For a couple of years, things were so good, even when things were still going wrong. This little boy had so much life in his smile, and he was so excited about everything. Me and my grandson did so much together. We took long road trips together, went to every amusement park, museum, national park, beach, and aquarium. I brought him everything he could ever want. My huge house was filled inside and outside with every toy imaginable, and my heart was filled with so many wonderful memories. Eli was just such a bright light after such a long dark lonely time that I thought would never end. He came at the time when I needed him the most, when I was ready to take that final step and commit to dying.

While enjoying Eli, finishing my BS in Criminology, and working on my MS in Criminal Psychology, I was beginning to relax a little bit. Life was getting so much better, although I was still in constant pain, and there was no peace in my home, I had learned to live with it. I had a well-paying job that I loved, working for the Sheriff's Department in the prison, and had many wonderful friends. Our house was beautiful with a nice pool, and I couldn't remember when things had been this calm. I thought the storm was over.

Life was good, but there was an emptiness still growing inside of me at the same time. I was very aware of the devil lurking behind every corner, and I waited for it all to be taken away again. Fear began to stalk me day and night, and I started to entertain it like I was seeing an old friend again. The devil was just waiting for the perfect opportunity, for me to show signs of weakness, so he could blindfold me and take me captive for years to come.

Then one day, that fear became reality. Fear gave birth to cancer. October 1, 2008. "You have breast cancer," the doctor said, but I really didn't hear him. My head was already spinning from knowing that this was the only thing he could say to me. My breathing seemed to have stopped the minute he walked into the room. After all, he called me into his office and told me to make sure that I brought someone with me. This was the only possible conclusion. He could have said "the sky is falling" and I would have known it was the same results: cancer. Now my fate was sealed.

DEATH AND MERCY

Cancer is the word that changes your life. It echoes in your mind for years. It shakes you to your core and stops everything. Until the doctor says it to you, you cannot understand the devastation it brings to your heart, especially when you are not walking with God. I had no idea. Any dreams of a future are erased. Life is shattered and unstable with so much uncertainty that you cannot move. By then, I had already been in a very dark place for 10 years. I figured that this would be the end of my horrible journey as I endured a slow sad death like my mom did. This was not the beginning of this Valley of the Shadow of Death, but I was certain it was the end.

Strength ran out the door and weakness overtook me. Happiness died and anxiety surrounded me again. One day I was enjoying what I thought was a beautiful life again finally, and the next, darkness swept through like a hurricane and destroyed it all; I just stood back and watched. It was as though I was encased in delicate beautiful stained glass and someone came and shattered it; shards of glass cutting me deep as it fell to the ground.

But I knew it was coming as soon as I felt that lump under my arm. This time it was different from all the other lumps I had had over the years. This time I knew. I had no intention of fighting this. I figured the devil had come to make good his promises of my destruction and death.

This appointment was after a series of tests and a bunch of phone calls, first telling me that all my tests were negative from a surgical biopsy and many scans on my breast. Because they saw two spots on my mammograms, and they only biopsied one, I had to endure a second biopsy, a barbaric stereotactic biopsy. That was a modern-day form of torture, where I laid on my stomach on a huge table with lots of machines around me. This table had a hole in it where my breast hung down into another machine that scanned it. Then the doctor inserted a thick large needle that took out chunks of flesh from out of my breast while I was awake and not medicated! Whoever created this machine should be put in jail!

Now, all of a sudden, I had breast cancer. The doctor never said he was sorry for the misdiagnosis he previously gave me. He never once felt remorse for telling me I was fine a month ago, when I was not.

So, I got up and walked out. My husband was trying to console me, but I had no idea what he was saying. It was as though someone had drugged me with depression instantaneously. Everyone laughed around me and acted as though the world did not stop for me. Did they not know I was dying? Did they not care? I knew I was not going to live through this because this was the exact evil that killed my mother ten years prior! I had already been through so many other diseases and traumas that I had little hope of living much longer, and I was sure my husband was glad of that. He had already endured so much with me that I was surprised he was still here. Years of instability, rebellion against God on my part, and hopelessness, had torn me apart from him.

A few days later, I told my family, not even being sure as to the treatment I was going to get, and not being able to answer their questions or fears. The first thing my oldest sister said was, "You're going to die!" which was the same reaction I had. But hearing her say it made me so angry because she had said it. I almost turned around and slapped her in my kitchen in front of everyone. She was and still is the drama queen of the family, and because of this, we were never really close.

For her to say this was a knife through my heart. I knew at that moment that I had to find a way to survive this to spite her. I had to fight. Once you get me angry, it's all over for you! I guess God had to use her fear and her uncontrollable mouth to wake me up.

I saw three different local surgeons and a few oncologists, and all of them had very different opinions on my course of action. They all wanted to cut me open right away, but yet they couldn't even tell me why or even remember my name. They all gave me very slim chances of survival, but yet they had no idea what stage of cancer I had or what type. Not knowing what else to do, I started researching everything on my own. I knew I had to find a place that knew what they were talking about. So, after some research online, I took all my records, biopsy slides, and scans, and went to a cancer research hospital, UCSD in La Jolla for a consultation.

When I drove up to UCSD, I was amazed. It was a huge hospital with valet parking, with lots of labs and student doctors. The beautiful buildings and gardens were like a resort hotel, and everyone was friendly and helpful. That first day, I met with three doctors, including the surgical oncologist, Dr. Blair, and a breast cancer oncologist, Dr. Schwab, and the head of plastic surgery, Dr. Chao. Dr. Blair stood out to me because she was so sweet and tiny, not even 5 feet, but so sure of herself. She was the David that stood before this giant in me.

When she came and talked to me, she pulled up her step stool and she stood there like a person on a mission. She gave me my choices and reasons. I was provided with so much information that I was overwhelmed. But she said we had time to decide and answered all my questions. She did not push me or scare me, but explained everything to me in detail, like she didn't have anywhere else to be, like she really cared.

Meditation Scriptures

Revelations 2:4-5 BSB

But I have this against you: You have abandoned your first love. Therefore, keep in mind how far you have fallen. Repent and perform the deeds you did at first. But if you do not repent, I will come to you and remove your lamp stand from its place.

Proverbs 18:14 GNT

Your will to live can sustain you when you are sick, but if you lose it, your last hope is gone.

Isaiah 30:15 NIV

This is what the Sovereign LORD, the Holy One of Israel, says: "Only in returning to me and resting in me will you be saved. In quietness and confidence is your strength. But you would have none of it.

Psalm 35:17 ESV

How long, O Lord, will you look on? Rescue me from their destruction, my precious life from the lions!

Psalm 43:3 BSB

Send out Your light and Your truth; let them lead me. Let them bring me to Your holy mountain, and to the place where You dwell.

1 Peter 5:8-9 NIV

Be alert and of sober mind. Your enemy the devil prowls around like a roaring lion looking for someone to devour. Resist him, standing firm in the faith, because you know that the family of believers throughout the world is undergoing the same kind of sufferings.

Joel 2:13 NLT

Don't tear your clothing in your grief, but tear your hearts instead. Return to the LORD your God, for he is merciful and compassionate, slow to get angry and filled with unfailing love. He is eager to relent and not punish.

Job 17:1 NLT

My spirit is crushed, and my life is nearly snuffed out.
The grave is ready to receive me.

Deuteronomy 31:5-6 BSB

The LORD will deliver them over to you, and you must do to them exactly as I have commanded you. Be strong and courageous; do not be afraid or terrified of them, for it is the LORD your God who goes with you; He will never leave you nor forsake you."

Psalm 68:19 NLT

Praise the Lord; praise God our savior! For each day he carries us in his arms.

CHAPTER 6:
BROKEN

"Even though I walk through the valley of the shadow of death, I will fear no evil, for you are with me; your rod and your staff, they comfort me."

(Psalms 23:4 BSB)

On January 6, 2009, I underwent a total mastectomy of my right breast with 10 lymph node dissection and a tram-flap reconstruction. They took my stomach fat and skin and reconstructed a new breast. This is the decision I made on my own. God had led me to this place, but I knew what surgery I wanted, never asking for His will for me. I was highly intelligent and believed I was making the right choice based on all my research. Besides, it meant I got a free tummy tuck at the same time.

This surgery was to be four hours and a few days in the hospital with a six-week recovery, but only a few days totally bedridden. I thought this would be a piece of cake! But, of course, things could not go smoothly. Because of so many complications during the surgery, it ended up lasting 12 hours, leaving me in ICU for seven days and in the hospital a total of 12 days. My body was so shocked and traumatized by this surgery that it fought back viciously. My arteries and veins, my heart, my breathing, my lungs, my blood, and my ribs were all complications that they had to deal with during this surgery, which I thought would be my only surgery for this, but I was so wrong.

When I awoke from the surgery, still groggy, I faintly heard a beautiful angelic piano playing, and I knew I must be in heaven. I made it! Suddenly, I became overwhelmingly sad because I realized I would not see my grandson anymore. Then the medication began to wear off. Reality hit hard; I was so nauseated and in so much pain when I woke up. The nurse kept telling me to push the button on the remote in my hand if I needed more pain meds. Every time I did, the morphine would pour into my IV, and I would doze off. But then I would stop breathing and wake up gasping for air. So, I fought for hours to stay awake because I thought I would die for sure. I would not push that button no matter how much I was hurting.

My chest felt as though it was crushed, and I could not breathe. I found out later it was because they removed part of my rib bone temporarily to reroute arteries from my stomach to my breast for blood flow. Lying flat for several hours with no pain medication, and being unable to move, caused my back and hips to cramp so bad that I could not stop crying. The only thing that kept me going was the need to see my grandson again. His face was all I needed.

The first few days in the ICU were terrible. People dying all around me, and family members crying, seemed like an hourly occurrence. They would bring whole families in to say goodbye and many got there just in time. That's what happens on a normal day in a cancer hospital. So much death and so little hope. So much heartache and so little life. So much sickness and so little of the presence of God, I thought. I could not imagine why God would allow this.

A few days later, they tried to sit me up time and time again, but I was so weak and sickly that it made me want to pass out. Unable to eat for days, I felt like I was getting weaker. I could barely move at all. Late at night, when my husband was gone, I laid there in tears. I felt hopeless because this was supposed to be easy, but it was not. Not for me anyways. I was supposed to be home by now, but there I was unable to think straight or move.

I wondered if God even understood how hard this was. How could He? Jesus never had a mastectomy! I wondered if I would get out of this hospital ever. Did they bring me to ICU because I was dying too like everyone around me? It sure felt like it. I wondered if I had made the wrong choice. Where was God? Why didn't He warn me?

I didn't notice how bad it was at first because of all the strong medications, but my thinking and memory were so damaged. My thoughts got so lost, and so often my mind was just blank. Believing this would wear off as they decreased the medication, I didn't let it bother me, but it just seemed to get worse.

On the 7th day, I was finally moved to a regular room. I was able to sit up and walk a few steps, but was still in a lot of pain. Not only in my chest, but also in my abdomen and back. Because of the nausea from the anesthesia, I was still unable to eat much. My right arm was extremely stiff, and I often got confused and disoriented.

Then one evening around 1:00 am, the nurse came to check blood flow in my new breast tissue with a handheld sonogram, and I had very little circulation. My skin was very cold to the touch, and she ran out of the room without explaining anything to me. Within an hour, my doctor was there, and they were wheeling me into an operating room, fear and uncertainty following close behind. The artery that they took from my stomach and redirected through my chest, used to supply blood to my breast, was constricted and my tissue would die without enough blood flow.

They took me into this small dark room with big machines and screens, and Dr. Blair got up on her big step stool and said they were going to use a heart catheter and balloon to open up the artery in my breast. They had never done this before and didn't know if this would work, but if it did not, they would have to surgically remove all of the new breast tissue right away. Because I knew what the heart catheter felt like, I began to panic; the thought of another surgery sent me over the edge. I could not endure another major surgery so soon, especially since I was still so weak. But this was the only option.

My husband had driven home 4 hours away, so he could not get back in time. I was so heartbroken and couldn't even speak except to say the name of Jesus as I lay there shaking. As I was staring at the ceiling with tears running down my face, a very large young man walked up to my side and took my hand. I noticed that he had the strongest and most gentle hands. His eyes were piercing and deep like that of a clear blue ocean, and a voice that was so powerfully peaceful. He said to me, "do not be afraid, I am always with you and I will not leave you." I've never seen anyone like him before or felt God's presence so strongly as at that moment in time. Immediately, the tears stopped, and I felt God's grace overtake me.

The procedure lasted only about 30 minutes. It was uncomfortable, but not too painful, and was successful. I went back to my room just so thankful to God for everything, especially for that man. Every time I went back, I looked for him at the hospital and asked who he was. Nobody knew who I was talking about.

Finally, day twelve, I was sent home. Not very strong, hardly walking, and hardly eating. But I was able to get up and use the bathroom with some help, which when you have been in bed for 12 days, it was my biggest accomplishment! I was grateful to God for that. Taking a shower instead of a sponge bath was amazing! And I just wanted to see my family and sleep in my own bed.

The nurse wheeled me to the car where Mario was waiting. I felt like I had been released from death row. So much weight fell off of me when I walked out of those doors, but yet I felt so broken. I was shaking so bad as all the emotion and fear left my body and mind. As we were driving off, my husband played "I still believe" by Jeremy Camp. I broke down sobbing like never before, so much pain so deep inside. My heart poured out all of my anguish. I was so shattered inside, and I could no longer hold any of it in. Tears flowed like a river, unstoppable and cleansing. He played this song over and over until I could cry no more. My heart was crushed, my soul was empty. And I was so grateful!

Healing was so slow, but I was home and my grandson's smile was all I needed. During the surgery, I had stopped breathing a few times. This, along with the effect of being under anesthesia for 12 hours, had caused so much damage to my brain. I was very foggy, confused, and at times very disoriented. A lot of short-term memory was gone! Once I was able to read a whole book each night, now I couldn't even read or comprehend a paragraph. I would watch a TV show and forget it all in a few seconds.

Remembering many things like details, names, places, or even major events was impossible. I had so much trouble expressing myself and would often forget what I was talking about in the middle of a sentence and never regain my train of thought. Trying to understand simple concepts was very frustrating for me. So many thoughts scattered in my mind. It was a constant battle to find my phone, my keys, my purse, and sometimes my house.

Oftentimes, I would lose myself, not knowing where I was or where I was going. This lasted for years. One day, I was trying so hard to remember my husband's name and it took me 30 minutes. Mario would call me "Fifty First Dates" and my kids called me "Dory."

Being home presented so many challenges for me. I had these four drain tubes attached to my body by painful stitches. The bloody fluid they collected had to be measured daily. I couldn't eat much of anything. Walking from one room to another could not be done without help, so Mario put chairs all around our long ranch style house so I could rest when going from one room to another.

With family far away, Mario had to take a lot of time off work to help me until I could manage being at home by myself. He had to do everything for me. My right arm was constricted because of the lymph nodes being removed, so the things we often do thoughtlessly were impossible for me. Oftentimes, it would freeze up so I could not move without excruciating pain. Brushing my hair or my teeth was very hard. Getting dressed was even harder. My arm would swell up with fluid and it was painful. Physical therapy did not help. The pain was never ending.

Most of all, the mental battles kept coming relentlessly: depression, loneliness, frustration, and mental exhaustion. These things, on top of confusion, made it seem like I was losing my mind. Each day, it felt impossible to go on. I would think of my mom and all that she went through. How alone she must have felt and how I did nothing to help her emotionally through these times. This terrible hopelessness and regret were overtaking me.

One thing about cancer or any major physical disease is you find out who your real friends are. I only had one. Everybody runs to help or at least say they will be there for you at first but soon forgets about you. Most people proclaim their love for you in public but are not there when you need them. This kind of love must be convenient and not cost them anything. This was so disappointing to me. The devil played on this far more than I had ever imagined, especially since I had always been there for others.

Meditation Scriptures

Psalms 138:7 NLT

Though I am surrounded by troubles, you will protect me from the anger of my enemies. You reach out your hand, and the power of your right hand saves me.

Psalms 119:71 NLT

My suffering was good for me, for it taught me to pay attention to your decrees.

Psalm 34:17-19 NLT

The Lord hears his people when they call to him for help. He rescues them from all their troubles.

The Lord is close to the brokenhearted; he rescues those whose spirits are crushed. The righteous person faces many troubles, but the Lord comes to the rescue each time.

Isaiah 30:18-20 BSB

Therefore the LORD longs to be gracious to you; therefore He rises to show you compassion, for the LORD is a just God. Blessed are all who wait for Him. O people in Zion who dwell in Jerusalem, you will weep no more. He will surely be gracious when you cry for help; when He hears, He will answer you. The Lord will give you the bread of adversity and the water of affliction, but your Teacher will no longer hide Himself—with your own eyes you will see Him.

Isaiah 42:16 TPT

I will walk[the blind by an unknown way and guide them on paths they've never traveled.
I will smooth their difficult road and make their dark mysteries bright with light.
These are things I will do for them, for I will never abandon *my beloved ones*.

Psalm 34:7 NLT

For the angel of the Lord is a guard; he surrounds and defends all who fear him.

CHAPTER 7:
NEVER-ENDING

"Lord, help!" they cried in their trouble, and he saved them from their distress.
He sent out his word and healed them, snatching them from the door of death."
(Psalm 107:19-20 NLT)

"The Lord is close to the brokenhearted; he rescues those whose spirits are crushed."
(Psalm 34:18 NLT)

Shortly after I came home from the hospital, my only son, Isaac, was getting ready to leave for Iraq for the first time. He was fresh out of Marine boot camp a few months prior, but I needed him home with me. I didn't know how I was going to let him go when it seemed like just yesterday I lost my baby son, Isaiah, who I never knew. In a wheelchair, drowning with tears, I sent him off to war. I will never forget how hopeless I felt at that moment as he boarded the bus and it drove away.

Fear was a heavy cloud over me releasing rain. I feared I would never see him again and it was unbearable. Each day, I sent him letters and care packages. Each day, I watched the news to make sure his unit was not hit. Each day, I prayed for God to be merciful. I felt God owed me that at least for all the suffering I was going through.

While living in fear of something happening to my son, little Dr. Blair had told me that they had biopsied all of my breast tissue they removed. From it, they not only found the two cancer spots we had known about prior to the surgery, but there were two other spots near my chest wall that had never been seen on any mammograms or CAT scans. She told me that I would have never felt these lumps. And if I were not being checked regularly, they would have spread beyond my chest wall and it would have been too late. I had had the choice in the beginning to just remove the two spots in a lumpectomy, but that would have been a huge mistake. That would have left the other two cancer spots free to grow undetected until it was too late. I was grateful for my decision.

Finally, 5 weeks after my surgery, the drain tubes were going to be removed. I was so happy, but I didn't understand how they were removed from my body or what it entailed. The stitches on my chest and abdomen where the tubes came out of my body, were so irritated and painful by this point that when the nurse touched them to cut them off, I screamed in agony. Each tube was pulled through the open incisions one at a time. This really freaked me out when I saw that there were at least two feet of tube inside of me at each drain site. It hurt inside and out, but mostly felt so incredibly weird like a snake inside of my body right under my skin slithering out. The nurse had described what she was going to do, but nothing could have prepared me for that.

After the tubes were removed, I went home happy to be free of those horrible things and ready to get better and back to normal. Unfortunately, a few weeks later, I saw a small sore on the side of my new breast on the incision. Over the span of a few days, it got bigger and deeper. I frantically called the plastic surgeon, Dr Chao, but he said it was nothing to worry about. By the time I got to see him a few days later, it had grown to about 1 inch wide, 3 1/2 inches long, and 2 inches deep. I was able to see into my flesh. He tried different types of washes and special bandages to close it, but nothing was working.

Eventually, he had me attached to this machine that draws the blood to the area to cause your cells to heal. The wound was packed with a special type of sponge and sealed with a clear surgical film, while this machine made embarrassing sucking noises the entire time. I had to wear that machine all day, every day, for 3 weeks, before the hole in my breast started to close. But then suddenly it stopped getting better. Thankfully, it wasn't getting any worse. The chance of infection was still so great, so I had to be careful.

A few weeks later, my doctor decided it was time to surgically close the rest of the opening. Back to surgery I went. More days in the hospital, followed by more horrible drain tubes, stitches that ripped my skin, anesthesia effects, horrible back pain, nausea, long recovery time, etc. This was just so unbearable. This was just so unreal. Every day I felt like I was suffocating.

To make matters worse, when the incision was repaired, it left me somewhat disfigured. Everything wasn't fixed. I still had a few other things that needed rearranging, so two more surgeries, many more days in the hospital, and many more complications. As well as the other torturous side effects, along with a few implants to even out my breast size. Afterwards, I thought I was finished.

Somehow, I survived, but I was very traumatized by the whole thing. I would joke that I had surgical PTSD, and it was true. Walking into the hospital made me shake with fear and I would cry. Watching medical shows was out of the question. Nightmares plagued me. I could not see anything traumatizing, like somebody falling down or getting hurt in any way, because I felt pain deep in my chest.

Despite the surgical PTSD I had been experiencing, I was surprisingly thankful to be alive. Suddenly, I wanted to live. From that time on, my whole perspective changed so drastically that I didn't know who I was anymore. Although there were still deep-rooted issues I was dealing with caused by all of this, I was just enjoying a reprieve from the never-ending storm. But that didn't last long.

One day, out of nowhere, my father suddenly got really sick. I was still on such an emotional roller coaster that this was really hard to handle. I couldn't breathe. At his age, 78, he was stronger than any 40-year-old, wiser than most people, lively, funny, extremely generous, and loved by all around him. He was the center of our world, and he made everyone feel like they were so special.

NEVER-ENDING

My grandson adored him, and my father never left my grandson's side. A few days before he died, my father was lying in bed unable to speak anymore or move, when my grandson crawled up in the bed beside him and snuggled with his papa. Tears began to fall down my father's face, and we all knew that leaving my grandson would be the hardest thing for him to do. I will never forget that day, the extreme sadness we all felt that has never gone away.

Within a few months, he was gone. I was in shock and disbelief, filled with a hollowing sorrow, wondering why this happened. He went peacefully on July 4th in the early morning, which was his favorite holiday of all. Later that night, while sitting in the back of the truck on a dirt road, while fireworks were going off above us at the local fairgrounds, we celebrated his life in silence, while our tears flowed freely. It is exactly what he would have wanted.

At my father's funeral service, several hundred people sat around his casket on a summer day singing "Amazing Grace," while doves were flying overhead. This knocked the life right out of me. As I sat on the grass under a tree with my grandson in my lap, I felt like I was being choked. I thought it should have been me in that grave. Honestly, I would have gladly traded places.

I felt pain beyond anything I had ever experienced. I was his little girl, his favorite, the baby of the family, and he was my rock. He had never failed me. How was I going to live now? I still needed him. Why would God allow this to happen to me after all I had been through? Had I not suffered enough for 10 people?

Years of 4-hour drives, appointments, scans, scopes, biopsies, and blood tests, making sure I was cancer free, followed. Accompanied with each new diagnoses; new tests, new procedures, and new medications. It never seemed to end. When listing all the diagnoses on any paperwork, in order to remember them all, I would have to start at my head. I would go through every part of my body downward, trying to remember what was wrong with that section of me.

As the years passed, everything was still very hard, but what got me through was the blessing of more grandbabies, including my two princesses and three more grandsons, and I got to see most of them come into this world. My love for all of them couldn't be any more fierce or deep, and it grew with every giggle, hug, and cuddle. Years later, things seemed to subside, I thought I was through all of the battles, and physically I was managing fine. But the damage to my emotions was so deep that even though we were making memories and growing, I was still dying inside.

The decay inside of me was still eating away at my heart. I had so many mental battles every time I looked in the mirror. I was ashamed of all my scars, the horrible disfigurement, the weight gain, and the ugliness that showed on my face. Feelings of worthlessness and bitterness plagued my brain day in and day out.

The only time I felt normal was when I was with my grandbabies. My appearance didn't matter to them. They eased my pain and made all the past disappear. All I had been through was forgotten when I saw their smiles. And they didn't avoid me when they looked at my face.

NEVER-ENDING

I knew people would avoid me because of my face. A "friend" once said I looked very rigid and harsh. That really broke my heart because they were not seeing my real heart. They did not look into my eyes. They did not hear my tears. They only saw the pain on my face and the torment I had endured from everything I had been through. The harshness from battles so long and fierce, that I barely survived, was evident in my expression. They could not understand and did not take the time to listen to my heart.

When I looked in the mirror, I would judge myself by what I saw. It crushed me. But I knew who I was on the inside, who I was destined to be. I often asked myself why couldn't anybody else see that? If they knew me for who I am, no matter what season or circumstance I am dealing with in my life, they would know that I am fiercely loyal. I would do anything for them, and I would fight for them. But that was all hidden away by the fortress of pain that surrounded me, imprisoning who God created.

Each day looking in the mirror was tormenting. It would make me so angry when I heard beautiful people talk about minor flaws. So superficial and vain. They were often too beautiful to lift a finger, too special to care about others, too concerned with their own beauty that they didn't really see other people. They had no idea what it meant to be flawed. They had no idea what it felt like to not feel like a whole woman anymore. They were so ungrateful for how blessed they were. I thought if they could spend one day in my body they would never complain again. They would be grateful for what they have.

I thought my body could not have been God's plan. Insensitive people would say, "you are made in God's image." But if they saw my body, they would know this is not what God intended. This all was so heartbreaking to me. After a while, my pain turned to anger, which planted so many seeds of bitterness.

Anger would rise in me when I would hear people complain about minor ailments or pains, when I could not remember a day without pain or even an hour. After seeing so many people suffering even worse than me throughout the years at the hospitals, I hated complaining myself. To hear people complain about minor stuff was an insult. They didn't understand what it was like to lose their hair, parts of their body, their minds, all their energy, and to live in pain 24/7.

If someone gave me an excuse why they couldn't keep their word because they had a backache or a headache, it would send me over the edge. How could people be so ungrateful for all the things working right in their bodies? They just didn't know what it was like to be me or the many hundreds of cancer patients I had seen suffering over the years. It made me feel like no one understood or cared what I had been through. These things were just too much to handle. All my emotions were extremely heightened during these years of torment, and they were unbearable.

I just wanted to be normal again, not beautiful, but normal. As I watched beautiful women, I was reminded of everything I was not. Feeling so ugly and unloved, and because I could not speak right, I withdrew even further from everyone around me.

During that time, I would have done anything to know that my husband still desired me. Instead of reaching out to him, I pushed him further away because of how repulsive I felt when I looked in the mirror. My insecurities devastated our relationship. There were so many things I did wrong, and at the time, I didn't care because I was the one who was suffering. He did not show me the understanding or compassion I wanted. He could not fulfill my emotional needs. No one on earth could.

It seemed like he failed me over and over again. But the truth was, it was me who was failing. I didn't see what he did for me. I couldn't appreciate how faithful he was to me and to God. I couldn't pay attention to him because I was barely surviving. Things just kept falling apart. We were ready to kill each other—literally. Two enemies living in the same house was hell on earth. Anything could have made me explode at any moment. Always trying to be happy on the outside just made me feel like I was going to crash on the inside.

Leaving Mario crossed my mind hundreds of times a day, but somehow, I stayed. I wanted him to leave me so he would not be stuck having to take care of me anymore. I felt as if I were a big burden for him, and that because of me, he missed out on his calling and so much of life.

As horrible as things were during this time, I was still content in my rebellion. I still did not want to go to church, even though I knew it was only because of God that I was alive. I wanted nothing to do with the hypocrisy, the loneliness, the emptiness of going to church with people that would look at me differently or would not love me back to health.

Driving down the road one day, I remember so clearly knowing that it was time. God was calling me very strongly, and I knew in my heart that if I didn't listen immediately, I would regret it. Still I would not surrender. And even though I was so far from God, He still showed me mercy despite my rebellion. His kindness and goodness bring us to repentance, but I was just determined to take the long road back home.

The problem with rebellion is that it has a ripple effect that could last for years. It affects everyone around us and can prevent even the next generation from realizing their own victories and destinies. In my case, I could not get victory over this evil that had tried to kill me for years, as long as I did not surrender to God. And therefore, my children and grandchildren would have to walk this same path until someone broke it. There is so much we miss out on when we hold on to our lives, even just a part of it.

NEVER-ENDING

Meditation Scriptures

Psalm 116:8-10 KJV

For You have delivered my soul from death, My eyes from tears, And my feet from falling.
I will walk before the Lord In the land of the living. I believed, therefore I spoke,
"I am greatly afflicted."

Isaiah 63:9 NLT

In all their suffering he also suffered, and he personally rescued them. In his love and mercy he redeemed them. He lifted them up and carried them through all the years.

Proverbs 20:6-7 NIV

Many claim to have unfailing love, but a faithful person who can find? The righteous lead blameless lives; blessed are their children after them.

1 Peter 5:10 NLT

In his kindness God called you to share in his eternal glory by means of Christ Jesus. So after you have suffered a little while, he will restore, support, and strengthen you, and he will place you on a firm foundation.

Psalms 18:6 BSB

In my distress I called upon the LORD and I cried to my God for help. From His temple He heard my voice, and my cry for His help reached His ears.

Psalms 119:76-77 BSB

May Your loving devotion comfort me, I pray, according to Your promise to Your servant. May Your compassion come to me, that I may live, for Your law is my delight.

Psalm 71:20

Though you have shown me many troubles and misfortunes, You will revive me once again. Even from the depths of the earth You will bring me back up.

Joshua 1:9 NLT

This is my command—be strong and courageous! Do not be afraid or discouraged. For the Lord your God is with you wherever you go.

Hebrews 12:15 AMP

See to it that no one falls short of God's grace; that no root of resentment springs up and causes trouble, and by it many be defiled;

NEVER-ENDING

Ecclesiastes 11:10 CSB

Remove sorrow from your heart, and put away pain from your flesh, because youth and the prime of life are fleeting.

James 1:19-20 TPT

My dearest brothers and sisters, take this to heart: Be quick to listen, but slow to speak. And be slow to become angry, for human anger is never a legitimate tool to promote God's righteous purpose.

Proverbs 31:30 TPT

Charm can be misleading, and beauty is vain and so quickly fades, but this virtuous woman lives in the wonder, awe, and fear of the Lord. She will be praised *throughout eternity*.

2 Corinthians 7:10 NKJV

For godly sorrow produces repentance leading to salvation, not to be regretted; but the sorrow of the world produces death.

CHAPTER 8:
REBELLION'S END

"I call heaven and earth to witness this day against you that I have set before you life and death, the blessings and the curses; therefore choose life, that you and your descendants may live And may love the Lord your God, obey His voice, and cling to Him. For He is your life and the length of your days, that you may dwell in the land which the Lord swore to give to your fathers, to Abraham, Isaac, and Jacob."

(Deuteronomy 30:19-20 AMPC)

One day, I met a couple of pastors visiting at my husband's church, Kem and Dara Gaskin. I was only there to take pictures of my husband getting his degree after years of schooling. They intrigued me, and I was drawn to them, although I tried to stay away. Peace and joy flowed out of them. They were so kind, and I instantly loved them, but I didn't want to. I wanted to run from them. Their beauty was not superficial but peaceful. I was sure they could see all the pain and ugliness in my heart, and they would hate me if they knew who I was, but they just smiled.

I had not seen these traits in Christians for years. As I introduced myself, I told them I was a photographer, and if they ever needed photos for any church events, I would be glad to assist them. What did I just say? I don't even know why I said that, and I wanted to slap myself instantly. I never wanted to shoot photos for churches. I just wanted to be left alone. I just wanted to love God on my own, in my own way, because I knew people, especially pastors, would try to suck me back into all the never-ending chaos of church life.

Meeting them was all in God's plan and his perfect timing. He can be quite sneaky at times. They happened to have an event at a local theater that next weekend and asked me to come shoot. This was so scary and exciting at the same time.

The event was very powerful, but I was not ready for anything more. I tried not to pay attention to the messages. I went on my merry way back to a life of "me" after that. Weeks went on, and the invitation they gave me to come to visit their church was harassing me day and night. Eventually, and reluctantly, I went, and I said I hated it. Walking in this church for the first time was so paralyzing, and I thought I might die just from the battle going on inside of my head.

I made up as many things as I could to complain about: the church was old, the worship was terrible, the bathroom smelled, the word was boring, the people were awful. I am sure at that point God was laughing at me because

I knew I belonged there. I was determined to enjoy having a tantrum all by myself. God quickly brought to mind the time my daughter Emily was kicking and screaming on the floor of Target when she was three. This was an infuriating daily occurrence. She was always a difficult child from the time she was conceived, and she prides herself in being difficult even now at the age of 32.

With everyone watching, I walked out of the front door of Target and left her there with her older sisters secretly watching out for her. I wanted to run, laugh, scream, and spank her, all at the same time. I was just done! I imagine God probably should have felt the same way, but He was patient with me for so long.

I swore I would never go back to that church, but I did time and time again. After coming and going for a year, not setting down roots, I still complained about it. I would not make friends, and I am sure my face scared people off anyway. No one looked beyond my pain and saw my longing for God at first. I was content being left alone, but was so lonely.

I came when I wanted and sped off as soon as I could run out of there unnoticed. Then God stepped in and said, "no more!" I knew at that point I was stuck there, and I was not happy in the least bit, but I decided to give it a shot. It was the least I could do for God for saving my heartbreaking life. Little did I know that my real life was yet to be saved. I was now in this place I needed to be but didn't know why.

During that time, my marriage was still a disaster, and my home life was horrible, but I kept going, and unwillingly decided to get busy doing whatever God wanted. I needed to get my mind off my problems. Then I met one of the Elders of the church, Desirie Canedos. I knew I was in trouble then and I wanted to run. Every word she spoke was like love and fire mixed together, piercing the repulsiveness in my heart, exposing the darkness, and uncovering who I really was. It was very hard to look at her or be around her in all my ugliness, and yet I was drawn to what I needed in her spirit.

At that moment, in that state, I was detestable, broken and miserable, but yet she didn't let this deter her. She was fierce like no one I had ever met, driven by the love of God, and told me the whole unsugar-coated truth. Day or night, no matter what, she gave me the word, prayed for me, and corrected me.

When she would ask me a simple question like, "How are you doing?" I tried so hard to hold everything in, but the pain and ugly truths of my heart would come pouring out, and when they did, I was being delivered from them. I spent so many meals in restaurants with her, crying as God was healing and restoring me. She showed me the path out of the darkness that had surrounded me for years, but sometimes it seemed like she was dragging me out by the hair while I was kicking and screaming. I needed this for so long. I couldn't walk on my own, but I knew one day I would. I knew one day I would fly. Pain was still radiating from my life. I was doing things that were harmful to my walk with God and my marriage, but she never gave up on me. She knew I wanted God.

I thought hard about making the decision to surrender to God all the way. I knew that if I was going to do this, I was going to do it all the way. So, as painful as things were when God was dealing with me, I welcomed the fire. The hotter the better! I wanted everything burned away. I wanted this death more than anything. I wanted to surrender my whole life. I wanted all of God. And then one day, I realized I had never really known Him, but I would not stop until I did.

Meditation Scriptures

James 4:8 BSB

Draw near to God, and He will draw near to you. Cleanse your hands, you sinners, and purify your hearts, you double-minded.

Ephesians 2:4-5 AMP

But God, being [so very] rich in mercy, because of His great *and* wonderful love with which He loved us, even when we were [spiritually] dead *and* separated from Him because of our sins, He made us [spiritually] alive together with Christ (for by His grace—His undeserved favor and mercy—you have been saved from God's judgment).

1 Peter 5:10 AMP

After you have suffered for a little while, the God of all grace [who imparts His blessing and favor], who called you to His *own* eternal glory in Christ, will Himself complete, confirm, strengthen, and establish you [making you what you ought to be].

Malachi 3:3 ESV

He will sit as a refiner and purifier of silver, and he will purify the sons of Levi and refine them like gold and silver, and they will bring offerings in righteousness to the LORD.

Psalm 27:3 CSB

Though an army deploys against me, my heart will not be afraid; though a war breaks out against me, I will still be confident.

CHAPTER 9:
THE RIVER

"Anyone who believes in me may come and drink! For the Scriptures declare, 'Rivers of living water will flow from his heart.'"

(John 7:38 NLT)

Once again, I came face to face with that same demon, breast cancer, in 2016. This time, the cancer was on the left side. This really threw me for a loop, it knocked the wind out of me. This time, I questioned God as to why. After all, I was now walking with him, serving him, and loving him. I did what he wanted, so why now? I thought I was free, but I never felt so defeated in my life. Death kept reminding me that my mother died after her second bout with breast cancer, so now it was my turn.

This shook my faith like never before. *I had to have answers for myself, my family, and for the devil. I had to have weapons that the enemy could not challenge.* But this was an uphill battle. Fear harassed me every waking moment, and oftentimes in my sleep—when I actually did sleep. There were no words for how disappointed I was or how this was tearing me apart inside.

I just couldn't comprehend why I was here again. Especially since I was now planted in a church where the worship was incredible; the word of God preached from the pulpit was rich, and the revelation that flowed from those that preached there was pure and strong. So in being surrounded by this river of wisdom and power, I could not comprehend why this enemy would be allowed to come at me with such force and with no opposition. I had to be unguarded or weak in areas that were crucial. As far as my own relationship with God, I read, I journaled, I prayed but it was still unfulfilling and unsatisfying.

One day, God started showing me a river, and showed me how I was standing on the bank of that river in the heat, but never drinking from it. I stood there watching the life-giving river flow past me, but was not partaking in it. I was dying of thirst, but I had to be the one to drink. Others could not do it for me. God did not just want me to drink, He wanted me saturated in His river. All the benefits were in the river.

This was a revelation that he showed me over a few months little by little. There is so much more to it, but one of the main points at that time for my story is that I was not in his river yet. I was standing on the side waiting for someone to give me a drink.

This river will either leave you on the bank thirsty, sweep you away if you are unprepared or disobedient, or give you life if you are flowing in that river. I didn't understand all this. But I knew if I wanted to live, I would have to live in that river of his Spirit. And I could only do that by trusting Him.

This time at least, I had back up. Now I had the faith warriors I needed in my life to help me fight this. People who I knew that knew how to pray, and how to believe. I was not equipped for this fight alone. I now had the help of Elder Desirie, Pastor Dara Gaskin (Momness), who spoke such earth-shaking words, and sung beautiful prophecies over my life with a love I had never experienced before. Elder Beatrice Murray (Queen Bee), who is a force to be reckoned with, a fountain of pure gold wisdom I had never seen. This mighty woman of God literally hugs the devil out of people through God's love.

My crazy joyous faithful friend, Tirzah Shambley, who sings everything with such power and authority that demons run when she takes the microphone, was also a tremendous help to me. She has led me through the most intense battles at the altar by her beautiful spontaneous worship.

They preached the uncompromising truth of God, but I had to find the truth for myself. I had to have my own weapons of warfare. I had to work out my own salvation. I knew God wanted me to stand alone with Him totally dependent on His spirit. I just didn't know how yet.

Still not understanding fully, I went running to the altar, and I begged and prayed that I would not have to go through the same things I did before, hoping that God was hearing me this time. Thinking my chances were better this time, I gave it all I had, but fear still stood by smothering me at times. Panic attacks would consume me and I was thinking about dying again. All these old demons were back in full force and multiplying, and they were relentless.

I was still missing something. It always seemed like something was on the tip of my tongue; that everything I needed was right on the edge of my spirit, but I could not see it or grasp it. It was as though God was telling me it is so simple, but for me that meant it was too complex for my brain. I was so confused and frustrated. So, I took a leap of faith and jumped in the river, desperate to pursue God even if it killed me.

Now, I was being swept away by the river and I couldn't stay afloat. When I jumped in the river, I still had very little understanding of who God was, so I was panicking trying not to drown instead of trusting Him. Still living in fear, that weight was overtaking me.

The same consuming and overwhelming emotions went with me into surgery in April 2016, and the same complications followed. Again, not really asking God, I chose this time to have a tissue expander put in along with the mastectomy of my left breast, so that later, I could have an implant placed under my muscle. That would mean only one more surgery.

This time, 20 lymph nodes under my left arm were dissected. Cancer was found in one of them. Again, my arm and shoulder froze up and I couldn't move it for months, breathing problems, long term anesthesia effects, and my IV ended up infiltrating, and I began to shake from all the pain medication being poured into my body. I was going into shock; 6 horrific attempts of putting the IV back in my foot, days and days in the hospital, severe back pain, tubes coming out of my chest, etc. etc. I experienced so much trauma, I thought I would never breathe again.

Again, my surgical wound opened up, causing fluid and infections to build up in my chest. They sent me back to the hospital to have a tube reinserted into my chest while I was awake to drain all the fluid. I would have lots of pain meds, but the thought of them cutting me open and inserting a tube into my chest while I was awake was more than I could handle. While me and my husband sat in the waiting area, he told me to listen for God's voice, to hear what God was trying to tell me at this moment. So, I quieted myself, prayed, and listened until God spoke.

I went into the procedure, but told them I just wanted them to do the ultrasound for now. Later, I would decide if I was going to have it done. From the ultrasound, they saw I had some infection and fluid building up in the hole in my chest that was about 2 inches deep, and my skin was not attached to the muscle. Feeling like God gave me peace about it, I told them I would not have the tube put in. I would go see my doctor and talk to her about the next course of action.

A few days later, fluid and blood were pouring out through the hole in my chest. The doctor decided that the best course of action would be to open up my chest again and wash out all the infection internally because the expander was under my muscle. Afterwards they then would surgically close it. If they had put the tube in without cleaning out the infection under my muscle and closing the wound, it could have caused the infection to spread everywhere. I would have still had the hole in my chest and had to have another surgery anyway. So, one more surgery. More pain, more complications, more trauma to my body, more painful IVs in my foot, more drain tubes, more scars, more of everything.

Although I had dodged the tube in my chest a few days before, I was still very afraid of what would happen next. I was so confused as to why this was all happening again. I couldn't shake the feeling that I was blind to something important. God was trying to tell me something simple, but I was just banging my head against the wall.

Meditation Scriptures

Psalm 27:14 MSG

I'm sure now I'll see God's goodness in the exuberant earth. Stay with God!
Take heart. Don't quit. I'll say it again:
Stay with God.

Matthew 10:28 AMP

Do not be afraid of those who kill the body but cannot kill the soul; but rather be afraid of Him who can destroy both soul and body in hell.

Hebrews 12:15 NLT

Look after each other so that none of you fails to receive the grace of God. Watch out that no poisonous root of bitterness grows up to trouble you, corrupting many.

CHAPTER 10:
SURRENDERING

"We can rejoice, too, when we run into problems and trials, for we know that they help us develop endurance. And endurance develops strength of character, and character strengthens our confident hope of salvation. And this hope will not lead to disappointment. For we know how dearly God loves us, because he has given us the Holy Spirit to fill our hearts with his love."

(Romans 5:3-5 NLT)

When people asked me how I was doing, I would begin to speak of the things I was going through. I started to tell them but would notice that they would interrupt me to change the subject or get on their phone. Many people would just tell me what I should be doing. Or that I was doing things wrong, when they had no idea what I was going through. All they really wanted was to appease their conscience by asking, but they did not want to hear my heart. That might require something from them, to actually walk in love, to take the time to understand. A few people reached out in true compassion and listened, not only to my words, but to my heart crying out.

So many times, quitting was all I thought about. "Just walk out the door and this will all go away," the devil would whisper to me. It was very tempting, but how foolish that would have been. Walk away from God and go where? Back to what? I knew what was behind me when I was alone and being tormented, it was horrific. Life without God was unbearable. I couldn't go back there. Besides, the devil attacked me viciously for decades when I was separated from God. So, how could I even for a second believe what the devil was saying now?

I had to go forward through what I knew would be a battle for my life. There was only one way this was going to end! One of us was going to be defeated, and it wasn't going to be me! I had to walk through this battle in victory! Anything short of that would not be effective, would leave me dead, and I knew it.

The question now was: How? Just walking around quoting scripture and mimicking Christian confessions was not working for me. And not only not for me, but I also saw very few people walking in victory over their situation. We often settle for circumstances and outcomes believing that these shortcomings are God's will. I knew this was not how it should be. God was trying to show me there was so much more to it, but yet it was simple.

SURRENDERING

Isaiah 43:1-2 AMP

But now, this is what the Lord, your Creator says, O Jacob, And He who formed you, O Israel,

"Do not fear, for I have redeemed you [from captivity]; I have called you by name; you are Mine!

"When you pass through the waters, I will be with you; And through the rivers, they will not overwhelm you. When you walk through fire, you will not be scorched, Nor will the flame burn you.

For I am the Lord your God, The Holy One of Israel, your Savior."

Thankfully, Elder Desirie and Elder Beatrice were always there, my 911's, my life preserver in this river until I could learn to swim. Even though they had never experienced anything close to all I had been through, they went beyond their own understanding and let the heart of God speak to me through them. Until we understand a person's journey, we cannot understand how deep their pain is, but that does not mean it should limit our compassion. We should be able to love the person before we know them and their pain. Not just out of pity or understanding of their trauma, but out of true grace and humility.

We never know if at the time we reach out to love someone, if that is a critical time for them. You don't need to experience these things to have empathy for someone, you just have to walk in love and obedience. Love is always a sacrifice, love is always an action, love plays no favorites, real love never ceases, and real love never makes excuses.

Many people love in word, but not in deed. We wait for the emotion of love to surface before we act. We pick and choose who to love. Many people would not love me because of my appearance or age, and that broke my heart, but yet it taught me so much. God's love revealed to us, brings a response of love through us. It will always seek others to love, no matter who they are or what they look like. It will always find others to love, no matter what we are going through ourselves. This is the true way of life.

So, I vowed at that time that I would always love people through physical battles, as well as mental battles—like I wanted to be loved, like Jesus loves us, in truth and in action. I would ask and I would listen without interruption or judgement. I would pray continuously. I would never disregard a person's emotions, trauma, or battles, and I would always be there, no matter what it cost me. I would never make excuses.

After 7 weeks of injections of saline into my chest port, the expander ended up failing, leaking into my body, and needed to be replaced, but I said NO. I wanted it out and to be done with all of this. So frustrated with my body, I decided to wait. I could not take it anymore, so I just continued to focus on God. At this point, I was sure I must be doing something wrong or not learning something. God was trying to teach me through all of this. I knew I was not going anywhere until I understood. I felt so alone and frustrated again, but I was also absolutely determined to find my answers.

My left arm and shoulder were in so much pain that I could not lift my arm very high. The physical therapist said my shoulder was almost frozen in place, and it would take months of therapy to get it moving again. That would mean 4 hour drives, 3 times a week, for about 4-5 months—lots of pain and soreness, and lots of pain meds. It seemed like everything I did, did not work. Still so frustrated, my mental battles were overwhelming. My strength and determination were dwindling.

One day, during worship, I was so crushed by all that was still happening to me. Standing there sad and in tears in the back of the church, I heard God say so quietly and powerfully, "**Just worship me**." So that is what I set my heart to do. There was really nothing else I could do. I had always really loved worship, but now it suddenly became a desperate need and my only focus as I opened my heart to love God, no matter what was going on around me.

Relentless in my pursuit to worship God, little by little, each time wanting to scream. I would crawl my fingers up the church wall until I was able to lift my arms to my Father. Each time, God's grace helped me to go higher than the last time. The higher my arm went, the farther in worship I went; the more I wanted to surrender more and more of my heart, the clearer his voice became. With my whole heart, I began to intently pursue God. Raising my hands in worship to Almighty God is a great privilege and a sign of complete surrender—now to the only one who deserves it, it is all I desire.

One day, standing in the bathroom after a shower, I looked at all my scars in the mirror. It was devastating to see how I had been so disfigured, but the damage was mostly on the inside. I counted each scar (21), some had been cut in the same place more than once. A weeping came pouring forth out of the deepest parts of my soul like never before. ALL the pain from so many years came rushing back to the surface, every emotion became real again. I crumbled onto the floor as God spoke to my heart and showed me all the times He was there with me through all the pain. Times that I didn't realize.

I was so consumed with my own battles that I could not see how He had stepped in so many times with grace and mercy.

I wept at all the life I gave up, living in defeat for so many years because of rebellion. I wept in unbelief because I could have avoided so much by obedience and surrender. I wept with repentance for the hurt I passed on, the wounds I caused. I wept in sorrow for the complaining I had done. I wept at the thought that no matter what I have been through, Jesus went through so much more.

His scars were much deeper, forged in love. He showed me every drop of blood I shed over the years, and yet Jesus poured out so much more. How could I be sad for what I had been through? How could I complain even though I still felt that what I went through was all in vain?

I was content to ignore all this heartache, but God was not. I knew there would be a day when I would have to open the door one by one to all those pains, traumas, and the sadness that I kept hidden away. And that God would want those skeletons cleaned out of my closet. That day was the beginning of it. He was revealing to me all that we needed to face together, all that He was going to do in me now. He was preparing me for this new battle, something so deep that only He could do.

Right then and there, I surrendered to Him everything. Every tear, every ounce of pain, every emotion—was all His now. I knew it would be a long road, but I knew who I could trust now. The love He poured out on me that day instilled in me a faith and a fearlessness to move forward, to fight for my soul, to let him heal me through and through.

SURRENDERING

Meditation Scriptures

Ephesians 5:2 NLT

Live a life filled with love, following the example of Christ. He loved us and offered himself as a sacrifice for us, a pleasing aroma to God.

John 15:12-13

My command is this; love each other as I have loved you. Greater love has no one than this, to lay down ones life for one's friend.

1 John 3:18 GNT

My children, our love should not be just words and talk; it must be true love, which shows itself in action.

1 John 4:16 NLT

We know how much God loves us, and we have put our trust in his love. God is love, and all who live in love live in God, and God lives in them.

Psalm 57:7 NLT

My heart is confident in you, O God; my heart is confident. No wonder I can sing your praises!

John 4:23 ESV

But the hour is coming, and is now here, when the true worshipers will worship the Father in spirit and truth, for the Father is seeking such people to worship him.

Zephaniah 3:17 AMPC

The Lord your God is in the midst of you, a Mighty One, a Savior [Who saves]! He will rejoice over you with joy; He will rest [in silent satisfaction] and in His love He will be silent and make no mention [of past sins, or even recall them]; He will exult over you with singing.

Psalm 59:16 (AMP)

But as for me, I will sing of Your mighty strength and power; Yes, I will sing joyfully of Your lovingkindness in the morning; For You have been my stronghold

And a refuge in the day of my distress.

Jeremiah 31:3 NLT

I have loved you, my people, with an everlasting love. With unfailing love I have drawn you to myself.

Amos 5:4 NLT

Now this is what the Lord says to the family of Israel: Come back to me and live!

CHAPTER 11:
BEHIND THE SCENES

"But because of your great love I can come into your house; I can worship in your holy Temple and bow down to you in reverence. Lord, I have so many enemies! Lead me to do your will; make your way plain for me to follow."

(Psalm 5:7-8 GNT)

During the next few years, God was speaking to me constantly, teaching me so much. I was hungry, restless, and fearless. I put the final surgery off again and again. I knew I was not ready yet, and besides that, I was far too busy. Grandkids, traveling, business, and ministry, just did not allow me time to dwell on the past. Honestly, it was all a way to change my focus instead of dealing with it.

At least that was my intention, but God was still working behind the scenes. He was using everything everywhere I went to teach me, to prepare me, and to change me. While He was healing so many deep wounds. This restoration was so peaceful and gentle. Many times in worship, He would overwhelm me with his great love, while quietly restoring my soul. This only happened because I had fully trusted him and surrendered my whole heart.

God is so amazing because I thought he was giving me all this revelation so I could share it with others. I was excited to share my testimony too, but that never happened. I still couldn't express my thoughts well anyway, especially in front of a group of people. My thoughts still got lost, and speaking was not very easy for me. Later, I realized I could not share all of these years of trauma and pain because I didn't have the victory yet. I didn't even understand why I went through this. If I would have spoken of my years of torture, it would have been a cry for pity at the time. What was I to say, "I have been walking in defeat for 20 years because I was rebellious and disobedient, and I suffered as a result? Hallelujah!" Who would want to hear that? Everything in His perfect time. It was all for me at that time.

Until the time came, I just kept going deeper, wanting more and more, and enjoying my life. And without me even knowing it, He was gently and lovingly healing me deeper and deeper, while instilling something so much more profound in me: Himself. The more of my life I surrendered, the more I was alive, the more of him lived in me. Little by little, the chains were falling off and the walls that imprisoned me were crumbling. Even by me sharing all of this with you in this book, each emotion, horrible detail, and trauma, I am becoming free.

Throughout all the time that I went to La Jolla for every appointment, surgery, scan, etc., I would often visit this nearby beautiful beach that was usually pretty deserted. There were so many magnificent cliffs and unique rocks and such blue skies. It was always sunny with beautiful bright white clouds no matter what the season. This was such a powerful place for me, an intimate place God set apart for us. Our secret place, where I shed many tears, where I poured out my heart to God, where I worshipped him, where He spoke so clearly to me. And every time I left there, I felt His overwhelming unshakable peace.

This is where He taught me so much about the depth of His love for me. I saw the vastness of His heart in that blue ocean. He revealed the power of His voice by the crashing of the waves. This is where He consumed me with His greatness, when He spoke to my heart and said, "this is an ocean of your tears, and I have saved every one of them close to my heart. This was enough to make me cry for days. How could God, so magnificent and glorious, love me this intensely? But I knew He did. Nothing was more absolute for me as his love.

As I experienced the fullness of His love, everyone was always telling me to pray all these scriptures, proclaim declarations over my life, and quote healing scriptures day and night. Over the years, I had seen some people do this and get their prayers answered, but for me it was not something that felt complete in my spirit. There was still something missing. It often seemed religious when I would do it. I would start, but felt like I was not on the right path and felt no power behind it. There was no understanding to back it up. He just kept emphasizing, *"Abide,"* to me.

Declaring the word of God in prayer is scriptural and effective, but I had to be confident in what God put in my heart to do. He kept emphasizing where those words were to come from. I could not just quote any scripture. I could not just study anything. It was as though I had to follow His exact footsteps.

It had to be precise. It had to be rhema (His Word). And when I was obedient to this, I could not only remember it, but I saw each word in the radiance of God's heart. It took on a life of its own and I could not stop meditating on these words. There was power behind every word He spoke!

So, people would ask me to pray, and I couldn't do it without stumbling through my words. Not only because I still had a disconnection between my brain and my speech, especially in front of other people, but stress and tension would make it worse. Besides, this was just not how I prayed. I couldn't ask for many things from God for myself during this time like other people could. All I wanted was Him. I did not constantly remind God of his promises. I did not claim things. I couldn't recite 20 minutes of scripture like everyone else.

Sometimes, it made me feel unspiritual, useless to the church, and unaccepted. When praying for others or situations in my private time with God, He led me to only worship Him in acknowledgement of who He is in that situation, in gratefulness, in assurance, in respect, and in my own words. All I could do was magnify Him in that circumstance.

Instead of doubting what God had me to do, I continued to follow Him instead of others. God impressed on me to study certain things, journal everything He told me and to listen carefully to His voice. He would bring up specific scripture in my spirit that played over and over in my mind, and I mostly worshipped Him in my prayer time. All that I could proclaim was about God and His goodness, His mercy, His love, His faithfulness, or whatever He put on my heart all day long everywhere I went. This living fountain of water was producing exactly what God wanted to do in me, and I felt like my prayers were much more effective.

As I was reading through my journals for the past few years, I realized that the answer was there in black and white, written by my own hand. I had done this unknowingly in a few major battles over the years, only praying and declaring what God spoke to me, but now it was becoming an absolute plan of attack that was required of me. Most of the time, God would just speak things directly to my spirit. Sometimes, it came during conversations when a specific scripture would spark my spirit. And other times, I would wake up with a song that would seem like it was alive in me and written for me. For the first time, I felt like I was on the right path. The more He taught me, the more the confusion lifted about this long 20-year battle, and the clearer His intentions were for me now.

During this time, I saw God move time and time again, bringing answers to situations I did not ask for or realize were a problem. Prayers were answered that I had not prayed for yet. And things on my heart that I didn't even acknowledge yet were changed. Situations turned around instantly, and faith was becoming a reality for me. He brought blessings that I did not imagine were possible. He was taking care of every little detail in my life when all my attention was on him and him alone. He not only did this for me, but for my kids and grandkids also.

Suddenly, in the fall of 2019, I began to feel so much doubt in everything He was teaching me. Because of things that were said to me, I began to question who I was, the voice of God, and my faith. This was a time of testing before the battle that would lead me to victory. The ground started to feel shaky, but I would not let go. God rose up in me and said, "You know my voice. Be confident in what I am telling you. Do not let anyone's voice change my words." That solidified everything, and when I regained my footing, nothing could shake me. I began to seek his voice even more. Hearing his voice was all I desired, and I looked for him to speak to me in everything . . . and he did!

Even as I am sitting here writing this, I want to run off and just praise Him. Tears are streaming down my face as I sing, "You are worthy." This makes it so hard to write, but he is the only distraction I allow in my life anymore. He is welcome anytime, and He surprises me with his sweet Spirit and his goodness over and over again. Even at this very moment, He is pouring out His love on me and delivering me, setting me free, and showering me with His loving kindness. I could not ask for a more perfect moment. There are no words to express what He is doing in my heart right now, who He is to me, or how He is loving me.

BEHIND THE SCENES

Meditation Scriptures

1 John 2:27 TPT

But the wonderful anointing you have received from God is so much greater than their deception and now lives in you. There's no need for anyone to keep teaching you. His anointing teaches you all that you need to know, for it will lead you into truth, not a counterfeit. So just as the anointing has taught you, remain in him.

Mark 12:30 CJB

And you are to love *Adonai* your God with all your heart,
with all your soul, with all your understanding and with all your strength.

Psalms 29:1-4 (NLT)

Honor the Lord, you heavenly beings; honor the Lord for his glory and strength.
Honor the Lord for the glory of his name. Worship the Lord in the splendor of his holiness.
The voice of the Lord echoes above the sea. The God of glory thunders. The Lord thunders over the mighty sea. The voice of the Lord is powerful; the voice of the Lord is majestic.

Psalms 147:11

The Lord favors those who fear and worship him with awe inspired

Reverence and obedience, those who wait for his mercy and loving kindness.

Psalm 91:14

Because he hath set his love upon me, therefore will I deliver him: I will set him on high, because he hath known my name.

Psalm 93:3-5 CJB

Adonai, the deep is raising up, the deep is raising up its voice, the deep is raising its crashing waves. More than the sound of rushing waters or the mighty breakers of the sea, Adonai on high is mighty.
Your instructions are very sure; holiness befits your house,

Adonai, for all time to come.

Psalm 29:3 CJB

The voice of *Adonai* is over the waters; the God of glory thunders, *Adonai* over rushing waters,

BEHIND THE SCENES

John 15:7-8 ESV

If you abide in me, and my words abide in you, ask whatever you wish, and it will be done for you.
By this my Father is glorified, that you bear much fruit and so prove to be my disciples.

Proverbs 18:20-21 BSB

From the fruit of his mouth a man's belly is filled; with the harvest from his lips he is satisfied. Life and death are in the power of the tongue, and those who love it will eat its fruit.

Psalm 19:14 TPT

So may the words of my mouth, my meditation-thoughts, and every movement of my heart be always pure and pleasing, acceptable before your eyes,
my only Redeemer, my Protector-God.

Psalms 1:2-3 BSB

But his delight is in the Law of the LORD, and on His law he meditates day and night. He is like a tree planted by streams of water, yielding its fruit in season, whose leaf does not wither, and who prospers in all he does.

Psalm 112:7

They will have no fear of bad news; their hearts are steadfast, trusting in the LORD.

John 4:14 CJB

but whoever drinks the water I will give him will never be thirsty again! On the contrary, the water I give him will become a spring of water inside him, welling up into eternal life!

Psalms 23:3 BSB

He restores my soul; He guides me in the paths of righteousness for the sake of His name.

Jeremiah 29:12-13 AMP

Then you will call on Me and you will come and pray to Me, and I will hear [your voice] *and* I will listen to you. Then [with a deep longing] you will seek Me *and* require Me [as a vital necessity] and [you will] find Me when you search for Me with all your heart.

Psalm 91:14-15

"Because he has focused his love on me, I will deliver him. I will protect him because he knows my name. When he calls out to me, I will answer him. I will be with him in his distress. I will deliver him, and I will honor him."

BEHIND THE SCENES

Matthew 6:25-33 ESV

"Therefore I tell you, do not be anxious about your life, what you will eat or what you will drink, nor about your body, what you will put on. Is not life more than food, and the body more than clothing?

Look at the birds of the air: they neither sow nor reap nor gather into barns, and yet your heavenly Father feeds them. Are you not of more value than they?

And which of you by being anxious can add a single hour to his span of life? And why are you anxious about clothing? Consider the lilies of the field, how they grow: they neither toil nor spin, yet I tell you, even Solomon in all his glory was not arrayed like one of these.

But if God so clothes the grass of the field, which today is alive and tomorrow is thrown into the oven, will he not much more clothe you, O you of little faith? Therefore do not be anxious, saying, 'What shall we eat?' or 'What shall we drink?' or 'What shall we wear?' For the Gentiles seek after all these things, and your heavenly Father knows that you need them all. But seek first the kingdom of God and his righteousness, and all these things will be added to you.

Psalm 46:10

Be still, and know that I am God! I will be honored by every nation. I will be honored throughout the world.

Ephesians 3:17-19 NLT

I pray that from his glorious, unlimited resources he will empower you with inner strength through his Spirit. Then Christ will make his home in your hearts as you trust in him. Your roots will grow down into God's love and keep you strong.

And may you have the power to understand, as all God's people should, how wide, how long, how high, and how deep his love is.

May you experience the love of Christ, though it is too great to understand fully. Then you will be made complete with all the fullness of life and power that comes from God.

Isaiah 48:17-18 BSB

Thus says the LORD your Redeemer, the Holy One of Israel: "I am the LORD your God, who teaches you for your benefit, who directs you in the way you should go. If only you had paid attention to My commandments, your peace would have been like a river, and your righteousness like waves of the sea.

Psalm 46:4 TPT

God has a constantly flowing river whose sparkling streams bring joy and delight to his people.

His river flows right through the city of God Most High, into his holy dwelling places.

BEHIND THE SCENES

Psalm 62:1-8 NLT

I wait quietly before God, for my victory comes from him. He alone is my rock and my salvation, my fortress where I will never be shaken. So many enemies against one man all of them trying to kill me. To them I'm just a broken-down wall or a tottering fence. They plan to topple me from my high position. They delight in telling lies about me. They praise me to my face but curse me in their hearts. Let all that I am wait quietly before God, for my hope is in him. He alone is my rock and my salvation, my fortress where I will not be shaken. My victory and honor come from God alone.

He is my refuge, a rock where no enemy can reach me. O my people, trust in him at all times.

Pour out your heart to him, for God is our refuge.

CHAPTER 12:
I AM BLESSED

"On the day I called, You answered me; And You made me bold and confident with [renewed] strength in my life."

(Psalms 138:3 AMP)

"Since we are living by the Spirit, let us follow the Spirit's leading in every part of our lives."

(Galatians 5:25 NLT)

Finally, the time came when God instructed me to have the final surgery. One call, and a few appointments, and everything was set in motion. December 20th, 2019, at 1 pm, I was to arrive at the hospital. It was several weeks away, and God was urging me to keep studying His faithfulness, His heart, His love, warfare, and victory. His Word was alive to me.

I knew I would have to trust him fully before I got rolled into the operating room. The surgery and the outcome were not my focus. It was only knowing him and all his characteristics. It was trusting Him and Him alone. Because I pursued Him for who He is, I no longer cared about the outcome of the surgery, and fear was not a threat any longer. Knowing who God is, with Him by my side, I was ready for anything.

So, I was set in my mind to leave all the details of this surgery up to God. I knew of all the things that have and could go wrong, but a few months back, He spoke to me and said, "Do not speak any other name over your life except the name of Jesus." I didn't speak of those complications or diagnoses anymore, and I certainly wasn't going to do it now.

With a new heart arrhythmia that had been harassing me for the last year, I would not call it by name. But God still assured me that I was to go ahead with the surgery. My surgeon was not so sure, so I had to have lots of specialist visits and heart tests first. Still, I was more sure of who God is, so I didn't hesitate.

I soaked up the Word of God, studied every detail of every scripture He gave me. I listened intently for His voice, and it became clearer and louder and more constant. He drew me closer and closer. This depth of intimacy was far more than I had ever experienced in my life, and it was beyond what I dreamed was possible. But I knew there was still much more.

I couldn't go without His presence, and if I stopped hearing His voice, I would immediately start praying and searching for him to speak to me. I would wake up singing praise songs that were bubbling up from my heart.

As I drove down the road, He would speak so many wonderful things, that I was often overwhelmed with joy. He was abiding with me and surrounding me. Like a new love, I couldn't get enough of it, or be apart from Him even for a moment. His love is joyous and fulfilling and I just wanted more.

Once the dam broke, a flood was inevitable! I believed I was now flowing in that river, led by His Spirit, and I was finally at that place where the river of God's presence was continuous and unstoppable. But God took me one step further and showed me that I was not just in that river, but that river was *in* me! The river of His love was exhilarating, life giving, refreshing, and revealing.

My daughter took me and my grandbabies to Orlando, Florida in November 2019 to ride on everything we could! We all had a blast and never wanted to leave. The fireworks were breathtaking; the lights were spectacular; the atmosphere was so magnificent; the rides were exhilarating, some of the most wonderful things we ever saw, but I longed to be alone in God's presence. I just wanted to hear God's voice because nothing in this world compares.

The final day, we were on the Avatar ride and it was so exciting, unlike anything we had ever experienced. I looked over at my daughter and my grandkid's faces, and they were lit up, laughing so hard and screaming! Those are the moments God gives us that last forever because of His immense love. Those are the moments He gives us to fight for. Then the most amazing thing happened, God spoke through me in the most powerful and glorious way I have ever experienced, and I said His words pouring out of my spirit, **"I am blessed, they are blessed!"** The most simple, yet profound words, He ever said to me! Needless to say, I was so consumed with God at that moment, and crying like a baby on the ride!

That proclamation from Him echoed in my spirit day and night, and I said it out loud often, knowing that my kids and my grandkids were blessed abundantly because of His love. Every time fear came at me, I stopped it in its tracks with that proclamation over my life, my body, and my mind. That proclamation anchored everything that He had been telling me for the whole year. I am blessed and nothing could change that ever. I am blessed by His presence. I am blessed by His voice. I am blessed by His faithfulness. All that He spoke to me was undeniable now.

A week before the surgery, I was home alone enjoying the quietness of my home, when I was startled by His voice whispering to me fiercely saying, "I will sneak up on you, I will surprise you, and I will surround you." That is exactly what He did. All that week before the surgery, God was suddenly all around me like the Tower of David in Israel. A few years prior, we had seen this tower in Jerusalem, firsthand. It's massiveness and strength really spoke to my heart. How could humans create such a place of protection? It looked impossible to penetrate those walls. God's love is much more secure than any earthly fortress or a thousand armies. When you are inside that love, there is no pressure from the enemy on the outside of the walls, there is no effect of the enemy's schemes.

Surrounded by His presence on every side everywhere I went, sometimes very unexpectedly, I was enjoying this immensely. I spent most of that time unable to speak much because there are not words to describe what was happening. Many times, I would be in tears in the store as He just suddenly overshadowed me. It was beyond overwhelming. He was unstoppable like a river overflowing its banks after heavy rains. Nothing could stand in the way of His Spirit!

Anxiety and fear were pacing outside of my fortress of peace, ready to attack the I moment I showed any sign of weakness. They were waiting for me to let them in. Knowing that this battle was critical for the rest of my life, the devil was relentless. But God! He was everywhere. He reminded me of the time He told me, "do not bow." Surrendering to fear was not an option, I would not bow to it. I already knew how this story was going to end, and so those words emanated in my spirit, *"I AM BLESSED,"* over and over.

Journal Entry 10/22/2018

The anxiety and fear have been stalking me ready to attack when I show any sign of weakness. They want to blindfold me and take me captive for years to come. They want to suffocate the life out of me. But then God's still small powerful sweet voice calms the deep treacherous waters, the storm brewing, the eminent attacks. "Do not bow," He says. I will not bow to fear. I will only bow to the Prince of Peace. I will not bow to anxiety. I will only bow to God, who has never forsaken me. I will not bow to the trauma of my past. I will only bow to the one whom my soul loves.

A few days before the surgery, Elder Desirie said to me in passing, "This time, it will be different." As she said that, my spirit jumped, like it was grabbing those words out of the air and burying them deep in my heart.

Every time, in everything He spoke, God was intricately preparing me for this battle, ordering my steps and leading me beside still waters.

Isaiah 40:31 AMP

But those who wait for the Lord [who expect, look for, and hope in Him] Will gain new strength and renew their power; They will lift up their wings [and rise up close to God] like eagles [rising toward the sun];

They will run and not become weary, They will walk and not grow tired.

Me and my husband were in a hotel room near the hospital the night before the surgery, and God was filling me up with His Spirit. Excitement rose up within me as I knew this was going to be a victorious day! I was journaling everything He said, and I just wanted to stay there in his presence forever. I slept like a baby and woke up ready, not wanting to run away, but ready to walk confidently into this battle. Almighty God was with me and I was never so sure of anything in my life.

Joshua 1:9 NLT

This is my command—be strong and courageous! Do not be afraid or discouraged. For the LORD your God is with you wherever you go.

Journal Entry 12/19/19

The night before my surgery, sitting up amazed at the sweet presence of God I experienced all day today. He surrounded me, overtook me, and consumed me with such a beautiful love that there is no denying I am His treasure. My faithful Father will not leave my side, but assured me over and over that I was not alone, that this time would be different. Those words bring tears to my eyes as I remember all the times He was faithful during this long journey when no one else was faithful. A journey that only He could understand, only He could carry me through. A victory only He could provide. His word had truly been a lamp unto my feet. God is wanting me to come higher, to hear His voice on a level of intimacy and obedience that is rarely seen anymore. All I want is Him, all I desire is His presence, His sweet word and His arms. My worship will always strive to be what He is worthy of. Today, tears of joy instead of anxiety because He is the living God inside of me. No other can ever do what He does in my heart. No one surrounds me with goodness like He does, I am so blessed I can hardly contain it. No words can explain the presence of God I am experiencing, a peace that I cannot comprehend, a love that no man can give. So so good, powerful, and sweet. Praise God for His abiding Spirit. Praise God for His faithfulness, for His love, for His mercy, for His grace. Only you, Lord, has sustained me all these years. Only you, God, have kept me hidden away from the evil that has tried to kill me for so long. Only you, God, walk me into victory.

My tears, my pain, and my heartache have set an anchor into the depth of God's goodness and mercy. It has taken me to a richness of worship that I will never retreat from, but only go deeper with. My life and my words will only be a praise unto God for His faithfulness throughout my years of torment, but mostly for who He is, for how wonderful He is, and because of His immeasurable boundless love.

Meditation Scriptures

Songs of Solomon 7:10
"I am my beloved's, And his desire is for me.

John 7:38 NIV

Whoever believes in me, as Scripture has said, rivers will flow from within them.

Psalms 84:2 AMP

My soul (my life, my inner self) longs for and greatly desires the courts of the Lord;
My heart and my flesh sing for joy to the living God.

Matthew 6:21 AMP

for where your treasure is, there your heart [your wishes, your desires; that on which your life centers] will be also.

Ephesians 1:3-4

Blessed be the God and Father of our Lord Jesus Christ, who has blessed us in Christ with every spiritual blessing in the heavenly places, even as he chose us in him before the foundation of the world, that we should be holy and blameless before him.

Isaiah 58:11 BSB

The LORD will always guide you; He will satisfy you in a sun-scorched land and strengthen your frame. You will be like a well-watered garden, like a spring whose waters never fail.

Isaiah 30:21 ESV

And your ears shall hear a word behind you, saying, "This is the way, walk in it," when you turn to the right or when you turn to the left.

John 10:27-28 ESV

My sheep hear my voice, and I know them, and they follow me. I give them eternal life, and they will never perish, and no one will snatch them out of my hand.

Psalms 61:2-4 BSB

From the ends of the earth I call out to You whenever my heart is faint. Lead me to the rock that is higher than I. For You have been my refuge, a tower of strength against the enemy. Let me dwell in Your tent forever and take refuge in the shelter of Your wings.

Proverbs 20:5 (MSG)

Knowing what is right is like deep water in the heart;
a wise person draws from the well within.

CHAPTER 13:
NOT THIS TIME

"My enemies did their best to kill me, but the Lord rescued me. The Lord is my strength and my song; he has given me victory. Songs of joy and victory are sung in the camp of the godly.

The strong right arm of the Lord has done glorious things! The strong right arm of the Lord is raised in triumph. The strong right arm of the Lord has done glorious things!

I will not die; instead, I will live to tell what the Lord has done."

(Psalms 118:13-17 NLT)

I had always in the past been crumbling under the immense fear on the drive to the hospital, in tears, and ready to scream. Every time, seeing the hospital made me choke up and struggle to breathe, oftentimes, panic attacks would follow. Each time, I would be in tears, shaking, and barely able to speak, as I could barely walk to the surgical floor, knowing what I would be facing.

Not this time! As we arrived at the hospital, my heart was surrounded with a supernatural peace. Every time it came up to my face, fear's sword drawn and ready to attack, I did not flinch at all, but proclaimed, "I AM BLESSED!" Immediately this fear vanished. This was no longer just a powerful God-given proclamation. This was now a violently devastating weapon that destroyed the enemy right where I had never ever had victory before. This was now a weapon that sent the enemy fleeing from me seven ways. This weapon cut off his head! This time, it *WAS* different!

Psalms 149:4 NLT

For the Lord delights in his people; he crowns the humble with victory.

As they prepared me for surgery, I was enjoying the songs that God had given me to listen too. Even while they were sticking my feet several times with big needles trying to get an IV, I was calm. Yes, it was painful but not like before. No longer did pain have an effect on my emotions. I was so consumed with God's goodness that I could not concentrate on the pain. That was followed by eight injections in my back to block my nerves, which was weird because I felt them in my arms and chest.

The pain was sometimes intense, but I was unafraid. Then off we rolled into the surgical room. Passing by these huge windows overlooking the serene gardens, this beautiful sunshine streaming in, I felt a deeper peace than ever before, a comfort, a joy, and a protection like a warm blanket over me.

Just a few hours later, I woke up, my throat a little scratchy, but I didn't have any pain at all! No IV in my leg, no uncontrollable nausea, no massive headache, no grogginess, no excruciating backache, no complications at all—and no painful catheter! Yes, God!!! Then I realized I would have to get up and walk very soon to use the restroom, but I knew I would be able to. I was so grateful to God that I kind of felt almost normal!

Usually, the first night was very rough after each surgery because of the intense pain all over my body, nausea, and inability to sleep, but this time I slept really well. I didn't even wake up when they came in every hour to check on me and take my blood pressure. Many times, I had been so miserable that first night, but this time I was comfortable and hungry. The nurse brought me Jello and soup and it was so refreshing.

Early the next morning, I was tired of the bed pans and said I wanted to get up. Everyone was pretty surprised, but slowly the nurse helped me to stand. I was able to walk a few steps to the bathroom. The next time I got up by myself! I was never so excited! I don't take those small things for granted ever, especially because after having 10 previous surgeries; this was the first time ever that I was able to walk the next day after surgery, only 15 hours later. That was a miracle to me! Usually, it took 3 days or more before I could sit up, or maybe take a step or two without passing out. Now I could move my arms! I could brush my teeth! I was praising God. I knew He would be faithful. I knew He was God Almighty.

After every surgery, anesthesia would affect me so badly, I would have nausea for days, vomiting, headaches for months, and be groggy after surgery for a few weeks to years. But this time, I ate a full meal the next morning and kept it down and I was very alert. Immediately, I opened my journal because I knew this time I could comprehend what I was reading. I rejoiced over all that God had spoken to me over the last year as it all began to make sense. I was able to read and write like normal. The surgeon had said to prepare for 3 to 4 days stay in the hospital, but I knew that morning it wouldn't be long.

The doctor came in before lunch, and said she was so amazed that I was doing so great. No issues with breathing, blood pressure, heart rhythms or blood levels during the surgery or now! My God is good! No need for any more monitoring; and since I was eating, going to the bathroom, and walking, she saw no reason to keep me. So, she sent me home!!! One night, less than 24 hours after my surgery, and I was out of there! Hallelujah!

This surgery was just as physically invasive as any of the past surgeries I had had, and I had never stayed less than 3 days, and to as many as 12 days previously. Even then, I could barely walk or move, and my blood pressure, breathing, and heart rhythm had to be monitored and controlled. Usually, I would be in a wheelchair for a few days because I was too sick or weak to walk, and used a walker for weeks, but not this time. They had cut into my chest on both sides and went down under my muscle, but I had no pain!

The anesthesia had no negative effects on my body or mind. This in itself is a miracle! This time was different! All I wanted was a juicy hamburger, and my bedroom sanctuary, where I could spend time with the lover of my soul. I even walked into the hamburger stand on the way home and endured the ride home, 4 hours with no problems, other than my husband's driving! God is faithful!

After surgery, as the days passed, God continued to surround me, and I got better fast. The drain tubes hurt a little bit, but were ready to come out in 7 days instead of the usual 4 to 5 weeks. I was able to go up and down the stairs in a few days and drove short distances in 10 days. My stitches did not open up, but healed so quickly.

Still overtaken by God's presence, it was hard to speak much for weeks. This was not because I couldn't think, but only because I was overwhelmed with Him. The doctor wanted me on complete bed rest for 6 weeks, but I was at church 2 weeks after the surgery, taking it easy and giving a short testimony in tears regarding His faithfulness. I would not wait six weeks to stand in worship before the altar for the one whom my soul loves! Even as I am writing some of this, 14 days after my surgery, I feel so great, almost normal, except for the random nerve pain in my chest as I heal, and also due to this compression bra that does not let me breath.

Meditation Scriptures

Psalm 23:6 KJV

Surely goodness and mercy shall follow me All the days of my life; And I will dwell in the house of the Lord Forever.

Isaiah 26:3

You will keep the mind that is dependent on You in perfect peace, for it is trusting in You.

Hebrews 10:23 AMP

Let us seize *and* hold tightly the confession of our hope without wavering, for He who promised is reliable *and* trustworthy *and* faithful [to His word].

Isaiah 9:2 KJV

The people that walked in darkness have seen a great light: they that dwell in the land of the shadow of death, upon them hath the light shined.

Psalm 145:5-7 ESV

On the glorious splendor of your majesty, and on your wondrous works, I will meditate. They shall speak of the might of your awesome deeds, and I will declare your greatness. They shall pour forth the fame of your abundant goodness and shall sing aloud of your righteousness.

Romans 8:37 NLT

No, despite all these things, _overwhelming victory_ is ours through Christ, who loved us.

Isaiah 12:3-6 BSB

With joy you will draw water from the springs of salvation, and on that day you will say: "Give praise to the LORD; proclaim His name! Make His works known among the peoples; declare that His name is exalted. Sing to the LORD, for He has done glorious things. Let this be known in all the earth. Cry out and sing, O citizen of Zion, for great among you is the Holy One of Israel."...

Psalm 112:4-8 ESV

Light dawns in the darkness for the upright; he is gracious, merciful, and righteous. It is well with the man who deals generously and lends; who conducts his affairs with justice. For the righteous will never be moved; he will be remembered forever. He is not afraid of bad news; his heart is firm, trusting in the Lord. His heart is steady;[a] he will not be afraid, until he looks in triumph on his adversaries.

Psalm 5:12 ESV

For you bless the righteous, O Lord; you cover him with favor as with a shield.

Psalms 18:1-2 AMP

I love You [fervently and devotedly], O Lord, my strength."
The Lord is my rock, my fortress, and the One who rescues me;
My God, my rock *and* strength in whom I trust *and* take refuge;
My shield, and the horn of my salvation, my high tower—my stronghold.

Isaiah 32:38-41 AMP

They will be My people, and I will be their God; and I will give them one heart and one way, that they may [reverently] fear Me forever, for their own good and for the good of their children after them. I will make an everlasting covenant with them that I will do them good and not turn away from them; and I will put in their heart a fear *and* reverential awe of Me, so that they will not turn away from Me. I will rejoice over them to do them good, and I will faithfully plant them in this land with all My heart and with all My soul.

Hosea 2:19-20 TLB

And I will bind you to me forever with chains of righteousness and justice and love and mercy. I will betroth you to me in faithfulness and love, and you will really know me then as you never have before.

Psalms 44:7 MSG

You're my King, O God— command victories for Jacob! With your help we'll wipe out our enemies, in your name we'll stomp them to dust. I don't trust in weapons; my sword won't save me— But it's you, you who saved us from the enemy; you made those who hate us lose face. All day we parade God's praise— we thank you by name over and over.

2 Corinthians 4:7-18 AMP

But we have this *precious* treasure [the good news about salvation] in [unworthy] earthen vessels [of human frailty], so that the grandeur *and* surpassing greatness of the power will be [shown to be] from God [His sufficiency] and not from ourselves. We are pressured in every way [hedged in], but not crushed; perplexed [unsure of finding a way out], but not driven to despair; hunted down *and* persecuted, but not deserted [to stand alone]; struck down, but never destroyed; always carrying around in the body the dying of Jesus, so that the [resurrection] life of Jesus also may be shown in our body. For we who live are constantly [experiencing the threat of] being handed over to death for Jesus' sake, so that the [resurrection] life of Jesus also may be evidenced in our mortal body [which is subject to death]. So *physical* death is [actively] at work in us, but [spiritual] life [is actively at work] in you. Yet we have the same spirit of faith as he had, who wrote *in Scripture*, "I believed, therefore I spoke." We also believe, therefore we also speak, knowing that He who raised the Lord Jesus will also raise us with Jesus and will present us [along] with you in His presence. For all [these] things are for your sake, so that as [God's remarkable, undeserved] grace reaches to more and more people it may increase thanksgiving, to the glory of [our great] God. Therefore we do not become discouraged [spiritless, disappointed, or afraid]. Though our outer self is [progressively] wasting away, yet our inner *self* is being [progressively] renewed day by day. For our momentary, light distress [this passing trouble] is producing for us an eternal weight of glory [a fullness] beyond all measure [surpassing all comparisons, a transcendent splendor and an endless blessedness]! So we look not at the things which are seen, but at the things which are unseen; for the things which are visible are temporal [just brief and fleeting], but the things which are invisible are everlasting *and* imperishable.

1 Peter 5:10 TPT

And then, after your brief suffering,[a] the God of all loving grace, who has called you to share in his eternal glory in Christ, will personally and powerfully restore you and make you stronger than ever. Yes, he will set you firmly in place and build you up.

CHAPTER 14:
HIS LOVE

"The LORD is a warrior; Yahweh is his name!"
(Exodus 15:3 NLT)

"For you are my hiding place; you protect me from trouble.
You surround me with songs of victory."
(Psalms 32:7 NLT)

As I reflect back to the day when I rolled into surgery, I thought I didn't have a full understanding of how this victory came into manifestation. I did not understand the season I was in now. I could not put into words everything that had happened and everything God had instilled in me. What God had required of me was faith and obedience: faith even when I didn't understand, and obedience without question. I walked into everything just simply trusting God, which is all He wanted from me. God gave me so much simple and profound revelation over the previous years, each step precise for me, but now I wanted to step back and see the whole picture in detail.

After I got home from the hospital, I asked God to teach me more details on how and why this time was different, and He had me write out, "The Spirit of a Warrior." It all came pouring out as He flooded my heart with everything that He had taught me over the last year within moments. He made sense of every detail and put it all into perspective, so that now I could see how it all worked together. Now, I started to see the whole picture. I could see those things that always seemed to be just beyond my comprehension, and they were all so simple. The battle plan was all in black and white in my journals, but it was not just for me anymore. I may not have understood all His methods or each step while I was going through it, but that was so I could put my faith in Him and Him alone. All He wanted was my unwavering "yes."

I knew that my faith was very divided and unstable before 2018 and that it would never get me anywhere. My heart was more turbulent than the ocean during a tropical storm. All my faith was planted in unstable and uncultivated ground. I had more faith in the disasters in my life than in the Deliverer, and more faith in death than in the Spirit of Life. I believed in the natural realm more than the supernatural reality. My knowledge of God far outweighed my revelation of Him, and my prayers went unanswered time and time again. I wondered why there seemed to be no power in my prayer, or only rare random manifestations of my faith. Not only for me, but for many others. So often I would hear, or I would say, "I am believing for . . ." Or hear/say prayers calling ambiguous things into manifestation, and it was as though something inside me repelled a lot of it, especially when I tried to claim or confess these things over and over. Rarely would I see results, but yet nobody could give me a reason why.

It was very confusing to me how Jesus spoke, and it happened right then and there. Some people Jesus never prayed for. He just spoke to them in specific words. He only said what he heard the Father say. He asked them questions confirming their faith and showing them how to declare the faith that was already inside of them.

The apostles all saw results with their own eyes, so why was I struggling even to get one answer from God for things He already promised me? What was faith? Why did it take forever? If we all got a measure of faith from God when we got saved, why did some produce a harvest, and many others did not? I needed to know this for myself as well as for others.

Hebrews 11:1 AMP

Now faith is the assurance (title deed, confirmation) of things hoped for (divinely guaranteed), and the evidence of things not seen [the conviction of their reality—faith comprehends as fact what cannot be experienced by the physical senses].

Hebrew 11: 1 EXB

Faith means ·being sure [the assurance; or the tangible reality; or the sure foundation] of the things we hope for and ·knowing that something is real even if we do not see it [the conviction/assurance/evidence about things not seen].

Hebrew 11:1 would play over and over in my heart, and I wanted that tangible reality, I wanted that faith foundation that could not be shaken, and I wanted to see the evidence in the spirit and also in the natural.

Everyone kept saying, "have faith," but nobody ever explained how. "Just believe," was not instilling *faith* in me but a *frustration* that would not stop.

I had always wanted to pray for people, especially for healing, but felt that it was useless when the same people were coming up for prayer time and time again, year after year, and healing was not being manifested. If many anointed preachers from all over the world could not get results, how could I? And why did people have to get delivered over and over again from the same thing? Yes, there were changes in some people, there were healings here and there, but manifestations were random, including in myself. How could I believe for others to get healed and delivered when I couldn't believe for myself? These questions plagued me day and night.

For so many years trying to do what I had been taught was frustrating to me. Even having the scriptures right before me, there was no flow, no peace in it. There always seemed to be something missing. There was just no true relationship with God to base my confidence in, and no anchor deep within my spirit to keep me stable in anything. I didn't know the heart of God, or the basic concepts of faith. I wanted answers for why I never received any manifestations throughout all these years. But what I sought after was still in the natural realm—knowledge and proof.

My faith was anchored in the flesh, the seen world, and that is an unstable foundation that obtains nothing in the spirit. Faith is not something that is as instantaneous as when you follow an instruction you receive from another believer to "just trust God." It is not a command that another human can impart to you. You will never have a faith with your mind that will produce any kind of results.

Faith was all that I wanted to pursue—the healings, the blessings, the miracles, and the gifts, but God said "no" each time, and led me in a different direction. And each time He changed my course, I turned around and walked back to pursuing these things again and again. That was just not where God wanted to take me right then, and I knew it. He was persistent in where my focus had to be. First, He had to change the desires of my heart, and I needed to let Him. I needed to desire Him and Him alone.

It was at that moment in worship when He told me, *"Just worship **me**,"* that changed everything for me. It was the fork in the road, the deciding point in my life to change my whole course. It altered my entire focus. He spoke these words gently and powerfully with love and authority, calling my spirit into alignment with his will for me, and calming the storm of unanswered questions. Worship was the cultivation of my heart, the breaking up of the ground that was so desolate, so that God could plant seeds that would produce a harvest of love, faith, and victory.

That was the first step down this path I took in complete obedience to His voice, but that step had to be *for* him and *about* Him. Nothing else. And I knew this the minute He spoke to me. It wasn't about my physical pain or the desperate need for Him to provide an answer. He was the path I was destined for, and although it was painstaking, it was so very worth it.

It was not a random command by God. He always has a divine purpose for everything He speaks. Everything He has ever done or said was for a precise season and reason. He did not give us thousands of scriptures just to say, "ok, now take all these scriptures and figure out the answer to your problem." No, He also gave us first and foremost, the Holy Spirit, to know

God intimately, and He has an exact objective in each of us, a path as unique to us as our fingerprints. The Holy Spirit is not dormant or there for us to just use when we are desperate—which I did for many years. When He is Lord over our whole lives, then we can be led down His paths for His purpose for His glory.

The Spirit of A Warrior
Who I am in Him!

A Warrior Spirit is not always fierce. She is the one that is undeniably changed in the presence of God, saturated with the unquenchable love by his spirit. She does not always roar but is softened by the gentleness and mercy of God that gives her unwavering confidence in a Father that defends her. There is bold fierceness in her quietness. There is immovable determination in her gaze. She has a spirit so open to the voice of God and allows her heart to be overwhelmed by the love her Father is pouring out. She is hidden away so deep in that love that she knows that no fear can separate her from him ever.

He pours this love out in the midst of battle as well as in the quietness of peace. He prepares a feast of his goodness and love for her, while the adversary cringes in the shadows knowing he is already defeated.

Her spirit believes nothing else except what her Father has spoken to her, his whisper stronger than any other voice, louder than the thunder, deeper than any ocean. She listens intently for his every word. She longs for his touch and is satisfied by no other. A love so much more real and consuming than anything she has ever known. His love is intense, relentless, faithful, and so gentle that it erases everything else from her mind.

HIS LOVE

She dedicates her sword to God, and lays down her own fight at his feet because she knows He fights for her and will never disappoint her. She lets him arm her with the perfect weapon for the storm. His promise of victory echos in her heart and she stands firm in that victory. A victory so sweet because it is shrouded in his love poured out in blood. A love she comprehends much more each day. A love that gives her boldness and confidence that she will not stray from or ever doubt.

This warrior anoints her King's feet with her tears, her broken heart she hands to him, knowing He is her strong tower, her defender, her redeemer, knowing that no tear was in vain but because she has poured out her heart to him, there is a faith like no other. No longer of fear, but tears of joy and gratefulness because of a love that brings strength and hope and peace.

He has turned her tears to wine. She has known a love that can not fail her, a perfect love. She walks into the storm knowing this love lives inside of her, abides with her, surrounds her and radiates from her. She sees every battle through that love. She sees who she is through this love. And she now sees others because of his love.

She closes her eyes and experiences victory within her heart. On her knees she is crowned with triumph by her King. Her Father places authority in her hands. He surrounds her with this power. He proclaims over her the defeat of her enemies long before the battle begins. She rejoices in worship, her faith confirmed in her shouts and in her whispers, and in dancing before her King as she carries the weapons he has given her right onto the battlefield. Sight does not deter her from running to the battle because she knows He will be there, He will lead her and He will be on the other side with her. Her only goal is to bring him glory, sing high praises, and testify of his goodness.

She walks into battle with her eyes closed led only by his presence, only listening for the sweet sound of his voice. When the battle is intense, she does not panic, but kneels in reverence for her Redeemer and keeps walking knowing this path was destine for her, knowing she can never be separated from his love. Faith is the only thing she knows. She can not fail. His love will sustain her forever. Darkness can not overtake her because there is a glorious light that comes from the Mighty Warrior within her, a light so purifying no evil can withstand it. His greatness is alive inside of her. No price too great to pay, no pain too deep to bare, she will always walk the path He lays before her knowing she is never alone, knowing He goes before her.

God has given her every weapon needed and as she is surrounded by her enemies, she is not moved because she knows the power behind these weapons. Every one of his proclamations of love are branded on her heart. She is armed with his immense love for her, the most powerful weapon of all. No matter what the battle, it does not stop the heart God has put within her to walk in love. As the fire refines her He surrounds her, and the enemy is consumed by the flames he sent to destroy her. What is left of her, is purity, precious gold, and is all God's.

She looks in the mirror at the many scars, wounds so deep from battles long and fierce, with tears in her eyes she thanks the Lover of her soul, her beloved one, knowing that not one of them was in vain and that they will never compare to the scars that Jesus bore for her. By his love He takes each piece of her brokenness and binds it back together like beautiful stained glass of many brilliant colors, a new strength that is only because of His deep and defining love for her He displays his new masterpiece in his kingdom for all to see. As His light shines through this new beauty, the glory of God is captivating and healing to others.

He stands over her a **mighty warrior**, knowing that what he has imparted to her has created a force to be reckoned with!

HIS LOVE

She now walks with victory in her hand, a weapon to defend herself and those walking through their own battles alongside her, those that are weary, those that do not yet know they are victorious. Only God.

Meditation Scriptures

Deuteronomy 20:4 NLT

For the LORD your God is going with you! He will fight for you against your enemies, and he will give you victory!

Psalm 23 NLT

The Lord is my shepherd; I have all that I need. He lets me rest in green meadows; he leads me beside peaceful streams. He renews my strength. He guides me along right paths, bringing honor to his name. Even when I walk through the darkest valley, I will not be afraid, for you are close beside me. Your rod and your staff protect and comfort me. You prepare a feast for me in the presence of my enemies. You honor me by anointing my head with oil. My cup overflows with blessings. Surely your goodness and unfailing love will pursue me all the days of my life,
and I will live in the house of the Lord
FOREVER

Jeremiah 20:11 BSB

But the LORD is with me like a fearsome warrior. Therefore, my persecutors will stumble and will not prevail. Since they have not succeeded, they will be utterly put to shame, with an everlasting disgrace that will never be forgotten.

HIS LOVE

James 4:7 NLT

So *humble yourself*s before God. Resist the devil, and he will flee from you.

2 Corinthians 10:3-5 NASB

For though we walk in the flesh, we do not war according to the flesh, for the weapons of our warfare are not of the flesh, but divinely powerful for the destruction of fortresses. *We are* destroying speculations and every lofty thing raised up against the knowledge of God, and *we are* taking every thought captive to the obedience of Christ.

Isaiah 54:17 BSB

No weapon formed against you shall prosper, and you will refute every tongue that accuses you. This is the heritage of the LORD's servants, and their vindication is from Me," declares the LORD.

Ephesians 6:10-18 CSB

Finally, be strengthened by the Lord and by his vast strength. Put on the full armor of God so that you can stand against the schemes of the devil. For our struggle is not against flesh and blood, but against the rulers, against the authorities, against the cosmic powers of this darkness, against evil, spiritual forces in the heavens. For this reason take up the full armor of God, so that you may be able to resist in the evil day, and having prepared everything, to take your stand. Stand, therefore, with truth like a belt around your waist, righteousness like armor on your chest, and your feet sandaled with readiness for the gospel of peace. In every situation take up the shield of faith with which you can extinguish all the flaming arrows of the evil one. Take the helmet of salvation and the sword of the Spirit — which is the word of God. Pray at all times in the Spirit with every prayer and request, and stay alert with all perseverance and intercession for all the saints.

1 Corinthians 15:57 BLB

But thanks be to God, the One giving us the victory through our Lord Jesus Christ.

Zechariah 4:6 NLT

Then he said to me, "This is what the LORD says to Zerubbabel: It is not by force nor by strength, but by my Spirit, says the LORD of Heaven's Armies.

Luke 10:19 NLT

Look, I have given you authority over all the power of the enemy, and you can walk among snakes and scorpions and crush them. Nothing will injure you.

Deuteronomy 28:7 ESV

The LORD will cause your enemies who rise against you to be defeated before you. They shall come out against you one way and flee before you seven ways.

Leviticus 26:7-8 NLT

In fact, you will chase down your enemies and slaughter them with your swords. Five of you will chase a hundred, and a hundred of you will chase ten thousand! All your enemies will fall beneath your sword.

HIS LOVE

John 16:33 WNT

I have spoken all this to you in order that in me you may have peace. In the world you have affliction. But keep up your courage: I have won the victory over the world.

Joshua 1:9 CEV

I've commanded you to be strong and brave. Don't ever be afraid or discouraged! I am the LORD your God, and I will be there to help you wherever you go.

Isaiah 42:13 NIV

The LORD will march out like a champion, like a warrior he will stir up his zeal; with a shout he will raise the battle cry and will triumph over his enemies.

Psalms 18:16-50 HSB

He reached down from heaven and took hold of me; He pulled me out of deep waters. He rescued me from my powerful enemy and from those who hated me, for they were too strong for me. They confronted me in the day of my distress, but the Lord was my support. He brought me out to a spacious place; He rescued me because He delighted in me. The Lord rewarded me according to my righteousness; He repaid me according to the cleanness of my hands. For I have kept the ways of the Lord and have not turned from my God to wickedness. Indeed, I have kept all His ordinances in mind and have not disregarded His statutes. I was blameless toward Him and kept myself from sinning. So the Lord repaid me according to my righteousness, according to the cleanness of my hands in His sight. With the faithful You prove Yourself faithful; with the blameless man You prove Yourself blameless; with the pure You prove Yourself pure, but with the crooked

You prove Yourself shrewd. For You rescue an afflicted people, but You humble those with haughty eyes.

Lord, You light my lamp; my God illuminates my darkness. With You I can attack a barrier, and with my God I can leap over a wall. God—His way is perfect; the word of the Lord is pure. He is a shield to all who take refuge in Him. For who is God besides Yahweh? And who is a rock? Only our God. God—He clothes me with strength and makes my way perfect. He makes my feet like the feet of a deer and sets me securely on the heights. He trains my hands for war; my arms can bend a bow of bronze. You have given me the shield of Your salvation; Your right hand upholds me, and Your humility exalts me. You widen a place beneath me for my steps, and my ankles do not give way. I pursue my enemies and overtake them; I do not turn back until they are wiped out. I crush them, and they cannot get up; they fall beneath my feet. You have clothed me with strength for battle; You subdue my adversaries beneath me. You have made my enemies retreat before me; I annihilate those who hate me. They cry for help, but there is no one to save them— they cry to the Lord, but He does not answer them. I pulverize them like dust before the wind; I trample them like mud in the streets. You have freed me from the feuds among the people; You have appointed me the head of nations; a people I had not known serve me. Foreigners submit to me grudgingly; as soon as they hear, they obey me.

Foreigners lose heart and come trembling from their fortifications. The Lord lives—may my rock be praised!

The God of my salvation is exalted. God—He gives me vengeance and subdues peoples under me. He frees me from my enemies. You exalt me above my adversaries; You rescue me from violent men. Therefore I will praise You, Yahweh, among the nations; I will sing about Your name. He gives great victories to His king; He shows loyalty to His anointed, to David and his descendants forever.

Psalms 144 BSB

Blessed be the LORD, my Rock, who trains my hands for war, my fingers for battle. He is my steadfast love and my fortress, my stronghold and my deliverer. He is my shield, in whom I take refuge, who subdues people under me. O LORD, what is man, that You regard him, the son of man that You think of him? Man is like a breath; his days are like a passing shadow. Part Your heavens, O LORD, and come down; touch the mountains, that they may smoke Flash forth Your lightning and scatter them; shoot Your arrows and rout them. Reach down from on high; set me free and rescue me from the deep waters, from the grasp of foreigners, whose mouths speak falsehood, whose right hands are deceitful. I will sing to You a new song, O God; on a harp of ten strings I will make music to You—to Him who gives victory to kings, who frees His servant David from the deadly sword. Set me free and rescue me from the grasp of foreigners, whose mouths speak falsehood, whose right hands are deceitful. Then our sons will be like plants nurtured in their youth, our daughters like corner pillars carved to adorn a palace. Our storehouses will be full, supplying all manner of produce; our flocks will bring forth thousands, tens of thousands in our fields. Our oxen will bear great loads. There will be no breach in the walls, no going into captivity, and no cry of lament in our streets. Blessed are the people of whom this is so; blessed are the people whose God is the LORD.

Psalms 91 BSB

He who dwells in the shelter of the Most High will abide in the shadow of the Almighty. I will say to the LORD, "You are my refuge and my fortress, my God, in whom I trust." Surely He will deliver you from the snare of the fowler, and

from the deadly plague. He will cover you with His feathers; under His wings you will find refuge; His faithfulness is a shield and rampart. You will not fear the terror of the night, nor the arrow that flies by day, nor the pestilence that stalks in the darkness, nor the calamity that destroys at noon. Though a thousand may fall at your side, and ten thousand at your right hand, no harm will come near you.
You will only see it with your eyes and witness the punishment of the wicked. Because you have made the LORD your dwelling— my refuge, the Most High— no evil will befall you, no plague will approach your tent. For He will command His angels concerning you to guard you in all your ways. They will lift you up in their hands, so that you will not strike your foot against a stone. You will tread on the lion and cobra; you will trample the young lion and serpent. "Because he loves Me, I will deliver him; because he knows My name, I will protect him.
When he calls out to Me, I will answer him; I will be with him in trouble. I will deliver and honor him. With long life I will satisfy him and show him My salvation."

James 1:6-8 NLT

But when you ask him, *be sure that your faith is in God alone.*

Do not waver, for a person with divided loyalty is as unsettled as a wave of the sea that is blown and tossed by the wind. *Such people should not expect to receive anything from the Lord. Their loyalty is divided between God and the world, and they are unstable in everything they do.*

Hebrews 11:16 MSG

It's impossible to please God apart from faith. And why?
Because anyone who wants to approach God must *believe both that he exists and that he cares enough to respond to those who seek him.*

HIS LOVE

Psalm 73:25 ESV

Whom have I in heaven but you? And there is nothing on earth that I desire besides you.

Psalms 42:2 NAS

My soul thirsts for God, for the living God; When shall I come and appear before God?

Jeremiah 29:13-14a NLT

"If you look for me wholeheartedly, you will find me. I will be found by you,"

Deuteronomy 30:19-20 NLT

"Today I have given you the choice between life and death, between blessings and curses. Now I call on heaven and earth to witness the choice you make. Oh, that you would choose life, so that you and your descendants might live! You can make this choice by loving the Lord your God, obeying him, and committing yourself firmly to him. This is the key to your life. And if you love and obey the Lord, you will live long in the land the Lord swore to give your ancestors Abraham, Isaac, and Jacob."

1 John 4:13 VOICE

How can we be sure that He *truly* lives in us and that we *truly* live in Him? *By one fact:* He has given us His Spirit.

Psalms 84:1-7 NKJV

How lovely is your dwelling place, Lord Almighty! My soul yearns, even faints, for the courts of the Lord; my heart and my flesh cry out for the living God. Even the sparrow has found a home, and the swallow a nest for herself, where she may have her young—a place near your altar, Lord Almighty, my King and my God.

Blessed are those who dwell in your house; they are ever praising youBlessed are those whose strength is in you, whose hearts are set on pilgrimage. As they pass through the Valley of Baka, they make it a place of springs; the autumn rains also cover it with pools. They go from strength to strength,till each appears before God in Zion.

Proverbs 20:5 HCSB

Counsel in a man's heart is deep water; but a man of understanding draws it out.

John 16:13 AMP

But when He, the Spirit of Truth, comes, *He will guide you into all the truth [full and complete truth]*. For He will not speak on His own initiative, but He will speak whatever *He hears [from the Father*—the message regarding the Son], and He will disclose to you what is to come [in the future].

Zephaniah 3:17 ESV

The Lord your God is in your midst, a mighty one who will save; he will rejoice over you with gladness; he will quiet you by his love;he will exult over you with loud singing.

Isaiah 40:31 NLT

But those who *trust in the Lord* will find new strength. They will soar high on wings like eagles. They will run and not grow weary.They will walk and not faint.

HIS LOVE

Ephesians 1:17-18 NLT

Asking God, the glorious Father of our Lord Jesus Christ, to give you spiritual wisdom and insight so that you might grow in your knowledge of God. I pray that your hearts will be flooded with light so that you can understand the confident hope he has given to those he called—his holy people who are his rich and glorious inheritance.

Proverbs 3:5-6 AMP

Trust in *and* rely confidently on the Lord with all your heart *And do not rely on your own insight or understanding.*

In all your ways know *and* acknowledge *and* recognize Him, And He will make your paths straight *and* smooth

[removing obstacles that block your way].

Psalm 5:7-8 NLT

Because of your unfailing love, I can enter your house; I will worship at your Temple with deepest awe.

Lead me in the right path, O Lord, or my enemies will conquer me.

Make your way plain for me to follow.

CHAPTER 15:
HIS LOVE LETTER

"Those who truly love me are those who obey my commands. Whoever passionately loves me will be passionately loved by my Father. And I will passionately love you in return and will manifest my life within you."

(John 14:21 TPT)

"But this is the new covenant I will make with the people of Israel after those days," says the LORD. "I will put my instructions deep within them, and I will write them on their hearts. I will be their God, and they will be my people."

(Jeremiah 31:33 NLT)

Late summer of 2018, God began to lay a solid foundation and expanded my understanding of Him. We had a 90-day bible challenge class at church led by Elder Desirie, where God specifically told me to study His love. At first, I resisted because I wanted to learn about faith and healing, but I knew I needed to be obedient. It began with me searching out the depth of His love for me, then He led me into learning how to love Him, and from there, how to love others. It blossomed into so many revelations of His Spirit. Never had I been so immersed in the depth of the Word of God as during that time.

The Word of God became alive, and I began to see it as a magnificent love letter. I was so consumed as God began to pour out His heart to me, and Him giving me so many opportunities to truly walk in love, and learning things I never knew about the details of God's Spirit, that I can't even express it in words. He was becoming absolutely beautiful to me and each word was precious to my heart. It was as though I was seeing a love story unfold before me that I was the center of. I began to know deep within me how truly special I was to God.

That fall, I went to photograph a women's retreat in Las Vegas for a local church. As I was walking around taking pictures during prayer and prophecies, I got cornered between chairs and people on the floor praying, I couldn't move. Then suddenly Prophetess Anita Scott, whipped around and looked at me straight in the eye with fire, out of so many women crowded around her. I tried to get away, but couldn't move without stepping on someone.

As she stepped out to walk toward me, it was as though the red sea of everyone around me parted and made way for her to stand right in front of me. She was truly a lion in the spirit, fierceness and fire poured out of her. When she looked at me, I was instantly overwhelmed with God's presence and power, like a tidal wave. She started to prophesy to me about many things regarding ministry, my life, and things that would come to pass, but then she said how very pleased God was with me, and that I was his beautiful treasure! She said that over and over again, barely being able to continue standing herself, with such excitement and fierceness, burning it into my heart!

Needless to say, I fell to my knees, overwhelmed, and overflowing with tears. I could hardly speak except to say, "Lord God Almighty, you are my beautiful treasure." I have no idea how long I was on that floor worshiping God, or what happened to my expensive camera, but I didn't care. God was so good that nothing else in this world mattered, but his voice. That's when I really truly understood in my heart what my focus had to be. My life had to always be intently focused on His words and His will alone. I knew instantly that God was confirming that He was to be my cornerstone, He was my treasure, and I needed to pursue Him relentlessly. I knew exactly what I wanted, and it was Him and Him alone!

Once I began to seek God's presence and voice, it all began to flow, slowly at first, and then like a flood. Journal after journal, I wrote everything down that God was telling me. Sometimes, He would be speaking so many things at once, I could not write them fast enough. Sometimes, it was one word, and other times, it was whole sermons. Still other times, it was so interesting, but I did not fully understand what He was saying yet.

Many times, it was a revelation that came forth step by step over weeks or months. Oftentimes, He spoke in parables showing me so much wisdom through things all around me. Sometimes, He would show me His wisdom in things from my past, revealing how He had had his hand on my life for so long. Much of it was so simple, but so powerfully illuminating for me.

Every time I drove on the freeway, He would speak to me, and there was nothing I could do, but soak it all in, even though I wanted to pull over time and time again. There were so many four-hour drives to La Jolla to see my doctors, that I don't know how I drove there! So immersed in God, it would seem like moments instead of hours. Later, I would try to remember everything He said to write it down, but oftentimes, I could not. I just had to trust God, it may not be accessible in my memory, but He was depositing things deep inside of me, these seeds that were hidden away until it was their time to spring forth.

Every word He said to me, every time, it came up from deep within me, an underground river that sprang forth to the surface, bubbling up, and producing such joy. Soon, it was a refreshing unstoppable waterfall overtaking me. I could not contain my tears. Sometimes, it was so extremely hard to drive when He surrounded me with His presence that I thought I might be pulled over by Highway Patrol!

Isaiah 58:11 BSB

The LORD will always guide you; He will satisfy you in a sun-scorched land and strengthen your frame. You will be like a well-watered garden, like a spring whose waters never fail.

Isaiah 41:18 KJV

I will open rivers in high places, and fountains in the midst of the valleys: I will make the wilderness a pool of water, and the dry land springs of water.

During this time, God brought such a clear understanding of what it means to wait on the Lord. Not only was I to wait for his direction in every situation, but I was to wait on his presence. I was also to wait for His precise word coming forth out of my spirit to instill the faith I needed and to renew my strength, to give me the courage to soar over any battle or situation going on below me. I was not to move until I heard His voice, and whatever He said to me was what I was to pray and stand on! The more I waited on God, the greater the strength was that I walked in. I sought after His voice in every moment, His presence in everything, and His heart in each detail of my life. In doing this, growing weary was not even a possibility. No longer was I struggling or toiling with my faith. It was beginning to flow and grow!

Over the next year, He took me further, my love grew and my desire for God's presence could not be quenched. His voice was springing forth in my spirit continuously as more things blossomed. I studied these words He gave me, and each one was so fascinating. He was abiding in me and with me. The rain of God came, and everything that laid dormant for so many years was beginning to bloom. It felt like a flood gate was beginning to break as I meditated on His voice. Waves of the Spirit of God began to overflow my life. More scripture came pouring forth from deep within me, more living water, more revelation. All I had to do was be obedient and wait upon His voice.

During the 90-day challenge bible class, as I began to study his love, I realized that for so long I misunderstood the love of God. He showed me that my knowledge of His love was so superficial compared to the revelation of His love that He was now giving me. For years and years, I tried so hard to grasp

His love with my mind, when it can only be realized with our spirits. I knew that there had to be more than what I had experienced, and what I had been told about, seeing it with my natural eyes, and by what I heard being preached, which was never satisfying to me.

For so long, I saw God through my own brokenness, my own past relationships, through my disappointments and my betrayals. I limited how much of His love I was willing to receive and how much love I was willing to give. God had to remove so much garbage from my heart, many weeds and rocks in my planting grounds, before my heart could even be cultivated to sow seeds of his love. These weeds were past hurts, traumas, all the suffering I had been through, errors in my thinking, faulty reasoning, and inaccurate teaching that had grown deep roots and spread turmoil throughout my life. They had destroyed my garden. Sadly, oftentimes, before we search out God and are delivered from our past, many Christians portray God's love to the world in a very distorted way, until we gain revelation; that was exactly what I did for so long.

Hosea 10:12 NLT

I said, 'Plant the good seeds of righteousness, and you will harvest a crop of love. Plow up the hard ground of your hearts, for now is the time to seek the Lord, that he may come and shower righteousness upon you.'

We humans naturally demand an exclusive love, a love that shows us we are most valuable to that person. Betrayal can end all of that in an instant and make the most beautiful thing in your life, ugly. It can change the need to love someone, and to receive love from them, to a passion of hate and vengeance. You can love someone with human love, and it can be lost over one sin. But God's love for us does not change because of a million sins.

My idea of God's love was like that of human love, like it is an act toward us, an emotion God has because He created us. Human love is simple, a feeling that begins one day and is often conditional or preferential. It can change because of our ever-changing emotions. When I thought of God's love like this, I was never satisfied in church or with my walk.

When we don't understand beyond our own reasoning the depth of His love, then we cannot be satisfied worshipping a God whose love we believe is as human love: temporal, emotional or conditional. Many in the church who have a hard time worshiping God openly, often have little revelation of God's love beyond their human understanding. It is not until we pursue and receive a revelation of His love that we will not limit how we worship or how we pray. This only comes from seeking Him and Him alone and denying what the flesh wants. God is so overjoyed to reveal Himself to us, we just have to want it! He wants to love us in ways we never thought possible, we just have to open ourselves up, despite all our past pains and betrayals.

1 Timothy 6:16 NLT

He alone can never die, and he lives in light so brilliant that no human can approach him. No human eye has ever seen him, nor ever will. All honor and power to him forever! Amen.

We can never comprehend the greatness of God and all He is through our natural minds and eyes. We can only receive more of the revelation of Him through our spirits. But we must have the capacity to receive what God is showing us of himself. God will not give us more than we are prepared for. He can only give us what we can contain, and we limit God in our lives in this way.

He spoke the word "capacity" to me in mid-2018 during worship, and I was under the impression He wanted me to serve more, do more, learn more. This was not what He was talking about. Later on, it became clear that He wanted me to expand my capacity for Him. My spirit in its present state literally could not contain the immensity of who God is. My soul was choking the life out of me, constricting my spiritual growth, so that had to change.

Matthew 9:17 BSB

Neither do men pour new wine into old wineskins. If they do, the skins will burst, the wine will spill, and the wineskins will be ruined. Instead, they pour new wine into new wineskins, and both are preserved.

We ask God for more of Him and yet refuse to obey His words. We are slow to follow instructions. We don't cultivate our own ground to receive it by spending time in worship, prayer, and the Word, and removing the things of this world. The seeds of this world expand your capacity for the things of this world and lead to death. The capacity for the great things of God cannot grow with fleshly desires ruling our lives.

1 Chronicles 16:9a NLT

HIS LOVE LETTER

For the eyes of the LORD roam to and fro over all the earth, to show Himself strong on behalf of those whose hearts are fully devoted to Him.

If He were to show me all the things He wanted to reveal to me at that time, it would have been like putting a river in an old wineskin. I would not have been ready to be saturated with him. Not fully understanding how this was done, I trusted Him enough to just say, "yes, Lord." I was determined to increase my capacity. I began to walk it out by just seeking Him even more in the areas He led me to. It was simple. I needed to replace those things in me that took up space, with more of God. I needed to be able to expand my real knowledge of Him and desire for Him, but I couldn't do this with so much clutter from the world. I just had to be obedient to every word and remove the unnecessary distractions and focus on Him. Everything unpleasant to Him began to fall off.

It was not always easy. I had to deny everything I had become. I had to relinquish all my ideas and knowledge, everything that had been rooted in my life had to die, and all that I had experienced in my past had to be forgotten. It took every ounce of strength at times, but God's grace was always accessible when I needed it. Many times, I did not dwell on the decisions I had to make, but just said no and never looked back.

I traded in my pain, for his presence. I traded in my tears, for His oil. I traded in my bitterness, for new wine. I traded in my own desires, for His desires. I traded in my own wisdom and understanding for the revelation of God. Slowly, the increase came. Slowly my capacity for the presence of God grew. Slowly, my desire deepened. And as I followed, step by step, He led me down roads of abundance and grace. For every ounce of my broken heart that I gave up, He gave me a double portion of mercy. For every physical limitation I denied in order to pursue him, He gave me triple blessings of his love. He was delighted in revealing more of himself to me every day, and I was overjoyed. He is all I wanted and yet I wanted more each day.

I had always held back part of myself and part of my life, but I could no longer do that. I always had a backup plan or a way of escape. Not anymore. It was all or nothing. God's plan was so much better. It was simple: just seek Him and He did the rest. Just obey, and He astounded me with His spiritual blessings. God was so relentless in revealing to me more about this love for me and how to open myself up to Him. If you want God and want to pursue Him, He will lead you, He will speak to you, and He will reveal who He is to you more and more each day. That is the deepest desire of His heart, that we desire Him.

On that day of the surgery, His love was perfected in me. His perfect love for an imperfect me, changed my imperfections into who He created me to be. Unlike the past 10 surgeries, and countless painful procedures and grueling tests, I had absolutely NO fear. It was just an empty emotion that tried to hit me from the outside like I was behind bullet proof glass, but it was no longer mine. This was a huge difference. I was seeing fear for what it really was. It was not in my head or my heart, choking the life out of me. I no longer feared the reality of my situation because I had a new reality!

Fear had no hold on me any longer, and that was God manifesting His love for me and in me because that is what He planted in me. That is what was bearing fruit now in the perfect season. All because now He was able to have full access to all of my spirit. All for His glory. All for me. All of it, so I could sit here and tell you the truth about God's perfect love for you.

Jeremiah 31:3 ESV

The Lord appeared to him from far away. I have loved you with an everlasting love; therefore I have continued my faithfulness to you.

God's love is the force behind Victory. When I sought to understand His love, my heart quickly understood victory because it is based solely on his love for us. Humility is the path to the river of life, and love is the power behind the river that overtakes us and brings us everything we need to overcome and live victoriously.

The bible describes God in many different ways. Many characteristics, yet they are all the same, all driven by a force of love so great. All of these aspects of God's love are not separate. Goodness, faithfulness, sovereignty, holiness, mercifulness, protection, etc., are all inclusive. Humans can operate in one emotion or maybe two at a time. But all of these things are not emotions in God but the whole essence of what God is. They are who He is, all at once, all the time.

1 John 4:8-10 & 16 NLT

But anyone who does not love does not know God, for God is love. God showed how much he loved us by sending his one and only Son into the world so that we might have eternal life through him. This is real love—not that we loved God, but that he loved us and sent his Son as a sacrifice to take away our sins.

We know how much God loves us, and we have put our trust in his love. God is love, and all who live in love live in God, and God lives in them.

John 15:9-10 MSG

"I've loved you the way my Father has loved me. Make yourselves at home in my love. If you keep my commands, **you'll remain intimately at home in my love***. That's what I've done—kept my Father's commands and made myself at home in his love.*

Ephesians 3:16-19 MSG

My response is to get down on my knees before the Father, this magnificent Father who parcels out all heaven and earth. I ask him to strengthen you by his Spirit—not a brute strength but a glorious inner strength—that Christ will live in you as you open the door and invite him in. And I ask him that with both feet planted firmly on love, you'll be able to take in with all followers of Jesus the extravagant dimensions of Christ's love. Reach out and experience the breadth! Test its length! Plumb the depths! Rise to the heights! Live full lives, full in the fullness of God.

His love will never change, and He cannot ever stop loving us, because then He would not be God. He cannot deny Himself. Everything else in this earth is subject to change but God's love! Love is who God is. He cannot be anything except love. His every action is out of deep unconditional love—every word, His presence, His power, because He cannot be anything else to those who belong to Him, except love. If only I had known this years ago!

HIS LOVE LETTER

Lamentations 3:22-23 GNT

The Lord's unfailing love and mercy still continue, Fresh as the morning, as sure as the sunrise.

Pure and perfect love that knows no bounds, that never fails. His love has no beginning and no end. His love is not predicated on who we are, but on who He is. His love is the only love that can bring transformation. His love is the only love that can restore us. His love is the only love that perfects us. It casts out ALL fear. And without fear, you will always have victory.

Mark 12:30 NLT

And you must love the Lord your God with all your heart, all your soul, all your mind, and all your strength.

His love is unstoppable. His love keeps our soul at peace, immoveable. His love preserves and restores our hearts. God's love heals us. God's love is not subject to disease, but disease is subject to God's great love for us. His love for us is mightier than all the rushing waters; it is quieter than the stillness of the morning over the deep, and more relentless than a torrential river crashing through dry land. There is nothing like it! Nothing on this earth compares, no beauty surpasses it, and no force can compare to its greatness!

Psalm 86:15 TPT

But Lord, your nurturing love is tender and gentle. You are slow to get angry yet so swift to show your faithful love. You are full of abounding grace and truth.

God's love is limitless. He uses great wonders of the world to show us the mighty things He can do. They are magnificent and they can overwhelm our minds by their beauty and greatness, yet his love is so much greater than all the goodness, beauty, and power in this earth. These things can be seen with our eyes, so they are limited, yet He has no boundaries, no limits, and does not hesitate to pour out His love on us. These things in the earth will pass away, but God's love never will. There is only a reflection of God in the things He has created. But in us, through us, it is God himself that can be manifested and is to be seen by the world. God has been poured out into our hearts.

Meditation Scriptures

Psalm 103:11 TPT

Higher than the highest heavens—that's how high your tender mercy extends! Greater than the grandeur of heaven above is the greatness of your loyal love, towering over all who fear you and bow down before you!

Psalm 41:11 AMP

By this I know that You favor *and* delight in me, Because my enemy does not shout in triumph over me.

Matthew 13:44 ESV

"The kingdom of heaven is like treasure hidden in a field, which a man found and covered up. Then in his joy he goes and sells all that he has and buys that field.

Matthew 6:21 TPT

For your heart will always pursue what you value as your treasure.

Proverbs 2:4-5 ESV

If you seek it like silver and search for it as for hidden treasures, then you will understand the fear of the Lord and find the knowledge of God.

Exodus 19:5 ESV

Now therefore, if you will indeed obey my voice and keep my covenant, you shall be my treasured possession among all peoples, for all the earth is mine;

1 Peter 2:9 TPT

But you are God's chosen treasure—priests who are kings, a spiritual "nation" set apart as God's devoted ones. He called you out of darkness to experience his marvelous light, and now he claims you as his very own. He did this so that you would broadcast his glorious wonders *throughout the world.*

Psalms 42:7 BSB

Deep calls to deep in the roar of Your waterfalls; all Your breakers and waves have rolled over me.

Isaiah 40:31 AMP

But those who wait for the Lord [who expect, look for, and hope in Him] Will gain new strength and renew their power; They will lift up their wings [and rise up close to God] like eagles [rising toward the sun];
They will run and not become weary, They will walk and not grow tired.

John 7:38 AMPC

He who believes in Me [who cleaves to *and* trusts in *and* relies on Me]

as the Scripture has said, *From his innermost being shall flow [continuously] springs and rivers of living water.*

Isaiah 12:3 AMPC

Therefore with joy will you draw water from the wells of salvation.

John 5:24 AMPC

I assure you, most solemnly I tell you, the person whose *ears [spirit] are open to My words* [who listens to My message] *and* believes *and* trusts in *and* clings to *and* relies on Him Who sent Me has (possesses now) eternal life. And he does not come into judgment [does not incur sentence of judgment, will not come under condemnation], but he has already passed over out of death into life.

Isaiah 55:11 AMP

So will My word be which goes out of <u>*My mouth*</u>, (rhema)
It will not return to Me void (useless, without result),
Without accomplishing what I desire,
And without succeeding in the matter for which I sent it.

Jeremiah 23:29 CJB

"Isn't my word like fire," asks *Adonai,*

"like a hammer shattering rocks?

1 Corinthians 2:13 NLT

When we tell you these things, we do not use words that come from human wisdom. Instead, we speak words given to us by the Spirit, using the Spirit's words to explain spiritual truths.

Psalms 1:1-3 NLT

Oh, the joys of those who do not follow the advice of the wicked, or stand around with sinners, or join in with mockers. But they delight in the law of the Lord, **meditating on it day and night.**

They are like trees planted along the riverbank, bearing fruit each season. Their leaves never wither, and they prosper in all they do.

Ephesians 2:4-5 AMP

But God, being [so very] rich in mercy, because of His great *and* wonderful love with which He loved us, even when we were [spiritually] dead *and* separated from Him because of our sins, He made us [spiritually] alive together with Christ (for by His grace—His undeserved favor and mercy—you have been saved from God's judgment).

Romans 8:37-38 BSB

No, in all these things we are more than conquerors through Him who loved us. For I am convinced that neither death nor life, neither angels nor principalities, neither the present nor the future, nor any powers, neither height nor depth, nor anything else in all creation, will be able to separate us from the love of God that is in Christ Jesus our Lord.

John 14:21 BSB

Whoever has My commandments and keeps them is the one who loves Me. The one who loves Me will be loved by My Father, and I will love him and reveal Myself to him."

Psalms 34:3-5 BSB

Magnify the LORD with me; let us exalt His name together. I sought the LORD, and He answered me; He delivered me *from all my fears.* Those who look to Him are radiant with joy; their faces shall never be ashamed.

HIS LOVE LETTER

Romans 8:14 AMP

For all who are allowing themselves to be led by the Spirit of God are sons of God.

1 John 4:18 NLT

Such love has no fear, because perfect love expels all fear. If we are afraid, it is for fear of punishment, and this shows that we have not fully experienced his perfect love.

Romans 5:5 AMP

Such hope [in God's promises] never disappoints *us*, because God's love has been abundantly poured out within our hearts through the Holy Spirit who was given to us.

1 Corinthians 13:13 TPT

Until then, there are three things that remain: faith, hope, and love—yet love surpasses them all. So above all else, let love be the beautiful prize for which you run.

Ephesians 3:19-20 TPT

Then you will be empowered to discover what every holy one experiences—the great magnitude of the astonishing love of Christ in all its dimensions. How deeply intimate and far-reaching is his love! How enduring and inclusive it is! Endless love beyond measurement that transcends our understanding—this extravagant love pours into you until you are filled to overflowing with the fullness of God!

Never doubt God's mighty power to work in you and accomplish all this. He will achieve infinitely more than your greatest request, your most unbelievable dream, and exceed your wildest imagination! He will outdo them all, for his miraculous power constantly energizes you.

CHAPTER 16:
GOD'S FAITHFULNESS

"Then Moses and the people of Israel sang this song to the Lord: "I will sing to the Lord for he has triumphed gloriously; he has hurled both horse and rider into the sea. The Lord is my strength and my song; he has given me victory. This is my God, and I will praise him—my father's God, and I will exalt him! The Lord is a warrior;

Yahweh[a] is his name!"

(Exodus 15:1-3 NLT)

Step by step, He led me further into the deep waters, adamant about me studying His love, His mercy, His grace, every trait of God, and finally for months, I was learning about His faithfulness. All I had to do was follow Him. This was when I felt like my faith really opened a door, like all those seeds began to spring forth and produce. I had a solid foundation of God's love, so now receiving revelation on His faithfulness was easy. It was as though I was finally wearing armor that was made just for me. This is when I began to see God for who He really is, face to face.

Faithfulness is the very core of how God operates and the anchor to our faith.

Journal Entry 1/12/2019

In this season, it is crucial to abide in the river. The sun will be scorching, and those that are not submerged in God will wither away faster than ever before. There will be no going in and out. We must remain in this hour. We must flourish in this hour, and we must pull others in before they wither and die. This living river, spoken word, the Spirit of God, must saturate every area of our life. It is a source for us, but also a source thru us for others. FAITHFUL rivers of all the promises of peace, wisdom, righteousness, health, salvation, prosperity, revelation, etc., flowing thru our hands, our spirits, our hearts.

Every verse I could find on His faithfulness I consumed. I worshipped Him for His faithfulness continuously, and very loudly proclaiming everything He was teaching me. He showed me so many times that He had been faithful over the years of suffering—in the big things but mostly in the little things.

When He sent me a nurse that took the time out of her busy schedule to massage my back for 45 minutes when I was crying in so much pain. When I met a lady on the elevator whose joy was contagious, even though she just found out she was terminal. When waves of peace would overwhelm me out of nowhere. When He was there during every dark night when my soul was crushed, and I cried alone. When my 3-year-old grandson, Matthew, walked through the halls of the cancer center waving and talking to everyone and brought so much joy and happy tears to so many sad and hopeless people. When He sent me beautiful vivid flowers, warm sunshine, and gentle breezes every time we were at the beach together. When my husband drove 4 hours each day to see me, and many times slept in the car when I was in the hospital. When I rejoiced with the lady at Costco when I told her I was cancer free, and she said she was also cancer free from ovarian cancer. When He gave me remedies and answers for chronic illnesses and problems I was having, and they disappeared. And when He sent friends and strangers with kindness time and time again.

His mercy carried me through every time. He was there with me all along. I just had to see it. Faithful! Even when I was blind to it. He was faithful even when I was not.

I had to see God for who He really is in order to change my outcome. I could not know Him by what I had been taught or from any preconceived ideas. He wanted for me to know Him intimately, and that cannot come from a 3rd party. My focus had to be fully surrendered to God in all aspects of my life—and most importantly, being obedient to His voice. It didn't matter whether it was in ministry or housework, giving or spending, serving, shopping, or being obedient to His voice in studying and prayer. I had to know who He was by His Spirit.

The proof of His faithfulness is not in what you see, but in what He says. These words stand true forever! His promises to us never change, and He has never taken back one word.

Psalm 119:90 AMP

Your faithfulness continues from generation to generation; You have established the earth, and it stands [securely].

Lamentations 3:22-24 MSG

God's loyal love couldn't have run out, his merciful love couldn't have dried up. They're created new every morning. How great your faithfulness! I'm sticking with God (I say it over and over).

He's all I've got left.

God's faithfulness was the final key I needed to understand, but I needed everything He taught me all year to complete the puzzle. He showed me that the faithfulness of God is absolute and can never change. Humans change their personalities, moods, and emotions, daily, and sometimes, hourly. We are swayed by everything around us and in us—past, present, and future. Our ability to remain stable is almost impossible at times.

Psalms 146:6 NIV

He is the Maker of heaven and earth the sea, and everything in them—he remains faithful forever.

God's attributes are not behaviors, and He does not only display these attributes outwardly toward us, but they are all of who He is—they do not change for any reason. God is faithfulness, God is love, God is mercy, God is healing, and every other attribute, and He cannot ever change. If God were not faithful, He could not be God. That is how absolute this is.

GOD'S FAITHFULNESS

Isaiah 54:10 KJV

For the mountains may move and the hills disappear, but even then my faithful love for you will remain. My covenant of blessing will never be broken," says the LORD, who has mercy on you.

Mount Everest would crumble, Niagara Falls would dry up, the sky would fall—all before God is unfaithful. This gripped my mind and awakened my spirit. He is so faithful that even when things appear as though they failed in the natural, such as in death, God can transcend our natural world, and He carries it forth in the spiritual world. Our sight is so limited by this world. We often limit our belief by what we can see, but that is not faith, and that does not mean God is not true to His Word. It is never going to happen.

He showed me that throughout the years, the goodness and faithfulness of God was not dependent on my circumstances. But my circumstances are determined by how I see His goodness and faithfulness, and by my obedience. It took me so long to learn this, always blinded by rebellion and pride when I could have spared myself years of torture. Just by knowing God, seeking God, obeying God, and wanting God, there is so much that He is restoring in my life.

Romans 3:3-4

True, some of them were unfaithful; but just because they were unfaithful, does that mean God will be unfaithful? Of course not! Even if everyone else is a liar, God is true.

PATRICIA SOTO

2 Corinthians 1:18-22

As surely as God is faithful, our word to you does not waver between "Yes" and "No." For Jesus Christ, the Son of God, does not waver between "Yes" and "No." He is the one whom Silas, Timothy, and I preached to you, and as God's ultimate "Yes," he always does what he says. For all of God's promises have been fulfilled in Christ with a resounding "Yes!" And through Christ, our "Amen" (which means "Yes") ascends to God for his glory. It is God who enables us, along with you, to stand firm for Christ. He has commissioned us, and he has identified us as his own by placing the Holy Spirit in our hearts as the first installment that guarantees everything he has promised us.

Before that moment, I often thought I was walking in faith for my answers, I believed for my healing, I believed for my miracles, but that faith was in word only—*my words,* not God's words. I quoted scripture until I was hoarse. I ran to the altar every time I had the chance, and I cried out to God for changes, and yet I was not obedient to His voice. I didn't even wait and listen for His Spirit. I didn't know who He was. I was doing it all in my own strength and knowledge. I didn't take His precise instruction seriously, even though I was hearing Him clearly at times. I know I did everything wrong for so long.

It took me forever to realize that I was constantly taking one step forward and two steps backwards. Always believing that doing good things in the flesh would result in spiritual progress. When we do things without the Holy Spirit's revelation and guidance, we are doing it out of our human nature which does not produce spiritual fruit—even when they are biblical principles.

GOD'S FAITHFULNESS

John 3:6 NLT

Humans can reproduce only human life, but the Holy Spirit gives birth to spiritual life.

When we ask out of our own motives, we open the door to manipulation, witchcraft, greed, lust, etc. We treat the word of God like a Magic 8 Ball. Never did God say He would be faithful to these prayers of the flesh, but only to His will.

Journal Entry 1/22/19

People are trying to use scripture to claim what they want, to prove to God He needs to do something for them, to manipulate the hand of God, and demand from God that which He already promised. We often use the word of God to fulfill the lust of the flesh. God is saying "No!" The Word of God is not a free for all, it is not a magic wand. When we allow God to reveal to us a word, His will, or a specific scripture through His Spirit for our situation or desire, it is a weapon of power, an assurance that it is God's will, faith evidence. It is the living Word of God that manifests His will.

James 4:3 NIV

When you ask, you do not receive, because you ask with wrong motives, that you may spend what you get on your pleasures.

Deuteronomy 13:4 NLT

Serve only the Lord your God and fear him alone. Obey his commands, listen to his voice, and cling to him.

Jeremiah 1:12 NLV

Then the Lord said to me, "You have seen well, for I am watching to see that My Word is completed."

2 Corinthians 4:13 ESV

Since we have the same spirit of faith according to what has been written, "I believed, and so I spoke," **we also believe, and so we also speak,**

Proverbs 18:21. AMP

The tongue can bring death or life ;those who love to talk will reap the consequences.

Life and death are in the power of the tongue. But what is driving your tongue? your mind? your flesh? or the Spirit of God? The second part of this scripture is never talked about. When we talk nonsense, we reap nonsense. Confession does not mean you believe. **It is when you hear what God is saying that you believe and confess. That is where power and authority lie.**

When we know the voice of God, our prayers and our lives will change! When we know the heart of God, we will desire and ask for those things that we know He wants for our lives. When our lives are about Him and not us, we will only desire more of Him.

God challenges our reasoning. Faith does not make sense, and sense knowledge doesn't make faith. I was looking at it all wrong for so long. I thought that faith was based on how I perceived things, my thoughts. I thought this mind-based faith came first, and then the manifestation would come next. Faith does not start with our thoughts and does not wait to see to believe. Faith hears with our spirits, speaks and sees the manifestation all together, all right now in the spirit.

Romans 12:3 NIV

For by the grace given me I say to every one of you: Do not think of yourself more highly than you ought, but rather think of yourself with sober judgment, in accordance with the faith God has distributed to each of you.

On my journey, He showed me how faith is from God. He was the one who planted the seed of faith in me. He was the one who cultivated it by his Spirit. He was the one who was giving the increase. He was the one who produced the harvest. I was just the ground—good ground because this is what I desired, He is who I sought after with all my heart. I was good ground because I said "yes" and meant it. I was good ground because I would not allow anything to shake me. And because I was obedient, His seed flourished in me when I meditated on it, searched it out, and confessed it. Faith came easy when these words came right from His Spirit to my spirit. The obedience came easy when I just wanted God and Him alone.

Hebrews 12:2 TPT

We look away from the natural realm and we fasten our gaze onto Jesus who birthed faith within us and who leads us forward into faith's perfection. His example is this: Because his heart was focused on the joy of knowing that you would be his, he endured the agony of the cross and conquered its humiliation, and now sits exalted at the right hand of the throne of God!

For years, I didn't know what to do with the Word of God. God showed me a man who had a basket full of seeds, and he treasures them because one day they would produce all he needed to survive. But he kept them hidden away. He knows every seed by name, how to plant and care for it, and what it produces, but He never plants them, never puts them deep in the earth, and then wonders why they do not produce anything. In time of famine, he wonders why he is starving. We take the word and do the same. We know the word and we treasure it, we memorize it, we recite it, but we never allow God to bury it in our spirit and produce what God wants it to produce in us. We never allow God to speak to us through it. We never allow God to prepare our ground.

What God said to me and revealed to me was life-changing to me because those are my seeds He has planted in my heart, the right seed in the right season. Not random seeds, but exact seeds for the coming battles. Not every seed is meant for every season. He already knew what I would be needing in my harvest for victory. God is always precise with what He does, that is why we must be precise in following His steps.

Those revelations that changed my life may not have any impact on you. You cannot produce a harvest of faith from seeds planted in someone else's garden. You have to have your own garden, your own seeds from the Father, and He will reveal to you the things He has destined for your life. But He can only do that if you seek him for yourself.

GOD'S FAITHFULNESS

Psalm 126:5-6 NLT

Those who plant in tears will harvest with shouts of joy. They weep as they go to plant their seed, but they sing as they return with the harvest.

We cannot live off of one harvest season. We must allow seeds to be planted in us continuously, so that we will have food for the rest of our lives. We must continue to be ready for each new seed planted, season after season, new gardens, new harvests, which produces seeds for the next season.

We cannot just walk in what we hear from many pulpits. We have to know God intimately. We have to know what God has for us individually. Our steps must be ordered, ordained, led by, and established by God. Only in that, will we not only have victory in every battle, but we will live in peace in the battle.

Meditation Scriptures

1 Peter 1:23 VOICE

You have been reborn—not from seed that eventually dies but from seed that is eternal—through the word of God that lives and endures forever.

2 Corinthians 9:10 BSB

Now *He who supplies seed to the sower* and bread for food will supply and multiply your store of seed and *will increase the harvest of your* **righteousness.**
Apostle Nathaniel Leon
"The Measure of your hearing, determines the measure of your faith."

Hebrew 10:23 NLT

Let us hold tightly without wavering to the hope we affirm, for God can be trusted to keep his promise.

Mark 12:30 NLT

And you must love the Lord your God with all your heart, all your soul, all your mind, and all your strength.

John 14:26 ESV

But the Helper, the Holy Spirit, whom the Father will send in my name, he will teach you all things and bring to your remembrance all that I have said to you.

John 6:63 ESV

It is the Spirit who gives life; the flesh is no help at all. *The words that I have spoken to you are spirit and life.*

GOD'S FAITHFULNESS

Psalm 32:8-9 ESV

I will instruct you and teach you in the way you should go; I will counsel you with my eye upon you. Be not like a horse or a mule, without understanding, which must be curbed with bit and bridle, or it will not stay near you.

John 15:7 NIV

If you remain in me and my words remain in you, ask whatever you wish, and it will be done for you.

1 John 5:14 NIV

This is the confidence we have in approaching God: that if we ask anything according to **his will,** he hears us.

Psalm 37:23 AMP

The steps of a [good and righteous] man are directed *and* established by the Lord, And He delights in his way [and blesses his path].

Galatians 5:16 AMPC

But I say, walk *and* live [habitually] in the [Holy] Spirit [responsive to *and* controlled *and* guided by the Spirit]; then you will certainly not gratify the cravings *and* desires of the flesh (of human nature without God).

Galatians 5:25 NLT

Since we are living by the Spirit, let us follow the Spirit's leading *in every part of our lives.*

Isaiah 55:8-13 NLT

My thoughts are nothing like your thoughts," says the Lord. "And my ways are far beyond anything you could imagine. For just as the heavens are higher than the earth, so my ways are higher than your ways and my thoughts higher than your thoughts. "The rain and snow come down from the heaven and stay on the ground to water the earth. They cause the grain to go producing seed for the farmer and bread for the hungry. *It is the same with my word.* **I send it out**, *and it always produces fruit. It will accomplish all I want it to,* and it will prosper everywhere I send it. You will live in joy and peace. The mountains and hills will burst into song, and the trees of the field will clap their hands! Where once there were thorns, cypress trees will grow.

Where nettles grew, myrtles will sprout up. These events will bring great honor to the Lord's name; they will be an everlasting sign of his power and love

Romans 8:5 GNT

Those who live as their human nature tells them to, have their minds controlled by what human nature wants. Those who live as the Spirit tells them to, have their minds controlled by what the Spirit wants.

CHAPTER 17:
HIS WORD

"For I am the Lord; I will speak the word that I will speak, and it will be performed. It will no longer be delayed, but in your days, O rebellious house, I will speak the word and perform it, declares the Lord God."

(Ezekiel 12:25)

The Word of God that the Holy Spirit brings to you, comes up from within your spirit. It is the faith seed that God planted inside of you, coming to maturity, and bearing fruit in the exact time God has specified. It is Him speaking to you and through you. God infused confessions! God infused faith!

When I started to see scripture in this way, from the point of God's voice speaking here and now, directly to my spirit, the Word of God took on a whole new direction and meaning. When I understood that the word "hear" means to actually hear with my spirit, and to "speak" only that which I hear my Father speak, and that the faith He planted in me is what God is saying precisely for this time, then faith became a whole new reality, and the Word became alive inside of me.

Ezekiel 12:25 ESV

For I am the Lord; I will speak the word that I will speak, and it will be performed. It will no longer be delayed, but in your days, O rebellious house, I will speak the word and perform it, declares the Lord God."

2 Corinthians 4:13 ESV

Since we have the same spirit of faith according to what has been written, "I believed, and so I spoke," **we also believe, and so we also speak,**

The key is to believe and then speak! Believe what God is saying to you right now through the Word, his voice, in your spirit, and speak that into existence!

There were so many scriptures that God spoke to me that I never remember hearing or reading. I had no scripture memorized any longer because my brain could not do that anymore. When my memory was lost, all the scripture was gone. It was so difficult to retain anything at all. The mind has nothing to do with the power of the spoken word of God. The power only comes through the Spirit of God.

When my memory was washed away, and my intelligence disappeared, it was such a blessing! No longer did I rely on my intellect, my own understanding or memorization, but only what my Father spoke to me. I had no choice, but to be led by the Spirit of God completely. The more I relied on Him for everything and listened for His voice, the more the Word became alive, and the more power was manifested, and as a result, my memory began to return. The fogginess lifted and He had more and more control of my spirit!

Hebrews 4:12 AMP

For the word of God is living and active and full of power [making it operative, energizing, and effective]. It is sharper than any two-edged sword, penetrating as far as the division of the soul and spirit [the completeness of a person], and of both joints and marrow [the deepest parts of our nature], exposing and judging the very thoughts and intentions of the heart.

This scripture I had heard so many times before, but when God spoke it to me, the emphasis was so different. He showed me that there must be a separation between the soul and spirit by the Word of God. These two can be so intertwined to the point that we believe that what we know in our soulish nature is our faith. Faith must be planted in our spirits through the Holy Spirit. The power of the word of God wants to infiltrate our spirits, which is the only way for the Word of God to produce a harvest, that is when it becomes effective in our lives.

Luke 8:12-15

Now this is the meaning of the parable: The seed is the word of God. The seeds along the path are those who hear, but the devil comes and takes away the word from their hearts, so that they may not believe and be saved. The seeds on rocky ground are those who hear the word and receive it with joy, but they have no root. They believe for a season, but in the time of testing, they fall away. The seeds that fell among the thorns are those who hear, but as they go on their way, they are choked by the worries, riches, and pleasures of this life, and their fruit does not mature. But the seeds on good soil are those with a noble and good heart, who hear the word, cling to it, and by persevering produce a crop.

In other words, we cannot plant seeds in our soul to grow a harvest in our spirits, but the harvest in our spirit can change our soul. Faith comes from the inside out. The seeds talked about in Luke 8:13 and 14 are seeds planted in our souls. Verse 15 is seeds planted in our spirit. Words planted in our soul can easily be washed away, but when we allow them to plant in our spirit, they cannot be uprooted.

When God breathes life to His Word, it is His power, His anointing, His fruits that flow through us. It is not in our own understanding or strength. It is His love that makes changes in our life, that ripens our fruit that changes our lives, so others can eat and be nourished. He is always wanting to do this for us and in us because He loves us.

The many fruits of the spirit are inevitable when in communion with God. Everything God touches reveals who He is, including our hearts. We cannot help but change and pour out who He is. When we are saturated, immersed in God, the things in our lives that are unholy, bow to the Spirit of God. But only when we make Him Lord. With love being God's primary characteristic, when that is evident in our lives, every fruit of the spirit easily blossoms and produces fruit that remains, so that others can eat and be fed.

Proverbs 4:20-22 NLT

My child, pay attention to what I say. Listen carefully to my words. Don't lose sight of them. Let them penetrate deep into your heart, for they bring life to those who find them, and healing to their whole body.

HIS WORD

Faith doesn't just fall out of the sky. *It comes from God,* and it requires an action on our part that we fully accept the living Word of God and live by it. God brings the mustard seed of faith when we say, "yes, Lord." Saying I believe, or I am believing for a specific thing, is not faith. Reciting scripture is not faith; it can be so religious if not done in the Spirit of God. The devil can quote scripture, and many people read the Bible with no manifestation of anything in their lives except religion.

I was so confused for 18 years, until I shut out all the voices and listened to His voice alone. It is what you speak and truly believe that will come to pass. When it is the voice of God speaking to me, I know it is already done. *The evidence and the reality of it is undeniable. His voice is that evidence.*

Hebrews 11:1 NLT

Faith shows the <u>reality</u> of what we hope for; it is the <u>evidence</u> of things we cannot see.

Matthew 21:22 ESV

And whatever you ask in prayer, you will receive, if you have <u>faith</u>.

Isaiah 55:11

So shall my word be that goes out <u>from my mouth</u>; it shall not return to me empty, but it shall accomplish that which I purpose, and shall succeed in the thing for which I sent it.

Mark 11:23

Truly, I say to you, whoever says to this mountain, 'Be taken up and thrown into the sea,' and <u>does not doubt in his heart</u>, but believes that what he says will come to pass, it will be done for him.

Matt 4:4

But he answered, "It is written, "'Man shall not live by bread alone, but by every word that comes <u>from the mouth of God</u>.'"

Matthew 17:20 AMP

He said to them, Because of the littleness of your faith [that is, your lack of firmly relying trust]. For truly I say to you, if you have faith [that is living] like a grain of mustard seed, you can say to this mountain, Move from here to yonder place, and it will move; and nothing will be impossible to you.

Luke 17:5-6

The apostles said to the Lord, "Increase our faith!" And the Lord said, "If you had faith <u>like a mustard seed</u>, you would say to this mulberry tree, 'Be uprooted and be planted in the sea'; and it would obey you.

The mustard seed is not the amount or size of your faith, but the immeasurable ability of that tiny seed God gives you to produce your faith—planted by Him in your good ground! A word, a verse, a saying, a song given to you by God Himself. This little mustard seed can produce a massive tree, just like the seed He gives you in your spirit will produce exactly what you need in a situation. It produces much more fruit than any other seed, so much fruit that you will be able to provide for others from the overflow.

Our faith is always there so that out of the overflow others can partake. And once the harvest from that seed is manifested, it will produce many more seeds to be planted for the next season! This faith is already available to us at any time and for any reason because the Holy Spirit is alive in us always!

Matthew 13:31-32

He presented another parable to them, saying, "The kingdom of heaven is like a mustard seed, which a man took and sowed in his field; and this is smaller than all other seeds, but when it is full grown, it is larger than the garden plants and becomes a tree, <u>so that the birds of the air come and nest in its branches.</u>"

Luke 8:5-18 NLT

"A farmer went out to plant his seed. As he scattered it across his field, some seed fell on a footpath, where it was stepped on, and the birds ate it. Other seed fell among rocks. It began to grow, but the plant soon wilted and died for lack of moisture. Other seed fell among thorns that grew up with it and choked out the tender plants. Still other seed fell on fertile soil. <u>This seed grew and produced a crop that was a hundred times as much as had been planted!</u>" When he had said this, he called out, "Anyone with ears to hear should listen and understand." His disciples asked him what this parable meant. He replied, "You are permitted to understand the secrets[a] of the Kingdom of God. But I use parables to teach the others so that the Scriptures might be fulfilled: 'When they look, they won't really see. When they hear, they won't understand.' "This is the meaning of the parable: <u>The seed is God's word</u>. The seeds that fell on the footpath represent those who hear the message, only to have the devil come and take it away from their hearts and prevent them from believing and being saved. The seeds on the rocky soil represent those who hear the message and receive it with joy. But since they don't have deep roots, they believe for a while, then they fall away when they face temptation.

The seeds that fell among the thorns represent those who hear the message, but all too quickly the message is crowded out by the cares and riches and pleasures of this life. And so they never grow into maturity. And the seeds that fell on the good soil represent honest, good-hearted <u>people who hear God's word, cling to it,</u>

and patiently produce a huge harvest. "No one lights a lamp and then covers it with a bowl or hides it under a bed. A lamp is placed on a stand, where its light can be seen by all who enter the house. For all that is secret will eventually be brought into the open, and everything that is concealed will be brought to light and made known to all. "So pay attention to how you hear. <u>To those who listen to my teaching, more understanding will be given. But for those who are not listening, even what they think they understand will be taken away from them.</u>"

Journal Entry 1/15/2018

The depths of his river we have not known yet, but He is taking us there. This river will flow thru the deserts bringing life to places that have been barren for years. It will feed the starving and water the withered. Nothing will stop it. It will expose the hidden things and destroy the things that are not of God. The river will cleanse those that want more of Him but will wash away those whose love is not true. We will go as deep as we want, but the deeper we go, the more freedom we have and the more life we receive.

Journal Entry 2/26/19

I have crossed over a threshold. Entered a new place I have never been before. New and Amazing. A clarity like never before in the spirit, where His words thunder and His voice echoes. It seems like color is alive and everything is a different dimension. <u>The Word was one dimensional before I came into this</u>

place. His voice was singular before I came into this position. Now it echoes in my spirit! *The power of God was unobtainable, faith was an illusion, and His presence was limited and at a distance. Now, I do not fear the intimacy. I do not question faith. It was never about seeking the healing, running after the calling, or chasing the blessing. It is and always will be only about God and Him alone. Nothing else matters and everything else matters. We must have a true uninhibited relationship, true bare intimacy, unashamed nakedness with God, a desire so deep we cannot deny it. I feel like I was blind before, not knowing true love, not completed and unfulfilled, until now. I was missing so much I never knew existed. I can never go back, can never cross that same threshold again, only forward, only more of Him. I only fear of doing without the presence of God. This keeps me from failure, keeps me from desiring anything of the flesh. An incredible thankfulness for this blessing breaks open my spirit even more every day. I just want more! It is as though the limits of my human capabilities have been removed, like I was constricted before, but now I can breathe deep. I have never been to this place, but I can never exist anywhere else again. The blessing is so abundant that I cannot contain it. And this is only the beginning.*

Now, finally, I was happy, I was at peace, and I felt his overwhelming presence every moment. I wanted more of God than I already knew about Him. I prayed often for more of his truth about Him. I spoke every God-infused proclamation over my life and over my kids every day! I was adamant about pursuing him and him alone.

There were several times when God said to me so clearly when I was lost in worship, "ask me anything right now and I will do it." Each time I would ask for more of Him, His voice, His wisdom, His presence. And He never withheld that from me. His Spirit would come in like a wave. I could have asked for a million materialistic things and I know He would have done it, but I know how temporal those things are, and that is not what I desired. There was only one time I asked for a situation to be resolved for my daughter, so that she would not have to have a major surgery to save someone else's life, and God was quickly faithful to his promise to me during that intimate moment.

God was showing me during the last months that faith must have an anchor in me. Faith's anchor is a revelation of who God is, the words He has spoken to you. For me, this anchor was the words He revealed to me through His spirit on His faithfulness for most of the year and the word, "victory." Each new word He spoke, building brick by brick, my faith. But the anchor I needed during the month of my surgery was what He spoke through me, "I AM blessed." He was not just blessing me. These words have been so engrafted in my spirit and have anchored my faith in who God is. It wasn't clear to me at first, but God purposely spoke strongly, "I AM," which is His eternal nature, the essence of who God is, Adonai, Yahweh! I AM blessed by God Almighty's presence! He could have said, "I AM," alone, and I would have been overtaken, but He went far beyond anything I could ask for and He called me blessed.

Mark 5: 25-34

A woman in the crowd had suffered for twelve years with constant bleeding. She had suffered a great deal from many doctors, and over the years she had spent everything she had to pay them, but she had gotten no better. In fact, she had gotten *worse. <u>She had heard about Jesus</u>, so she came up behind him through the crowd and touched his robe. For she thought to herself, "If I can just touch his robe, <u>I will be healed</u>." Immediately the bleeding stopped, and she could feel in her body that she had been healed of her terrible condition. Jesus realized at once that healing power had gone out from him, so he turned around in the crowd and asked, "Who touched my robe?" His disciples said to him, "Look at this crowd pressing around you. How can you ask, 'Who touched me?'"*

But he kept on looking around to see who had done it. Then the frightened woman, trembling at the realization of what had happened to her, came and fell to her knees in front of him and told him what she had done. And he said to her, "Daughter, your faith has made you well. Go in peace. Your suffering is over."

There were many miracles in the Bible God spoke to me through, but the one that impacted my faith the most was this little woman who had extreme faith. There is far more to the story of the woman with the issue of blood than we read. There are things only God can show you. God had me meditate on this miracle for many weeks, and He enlightened me to the depth of her faith. It was beautiful. She was considered unclean and untouchable, and anyone or anything she touched would be considered unclean. She suffered and was in agony by this physical ailment for so long. She was kept isolated, not allowed to be in public or go to the temple to pray. She was an outcast. I can imagine the loneliness and frustration that must have tormented her day and night for years and years, but she put everything aside. She did not let self-pity consume her.

The moment she *heard* about Jesus, she believed. It was her spirit that heard, not her ears. She proclaimed her faith, "if I can just touch his robe, I will be healed." Her faith was anchored, and she acted on that faith immediately without hesitation. And she had that unshakable mustard seed faith, and she knew He was her only hope.

The risk of being stoned for breaking the religious laws by going into public when she was unclean was great. But despite all of this, she not only went in public, *but she also pursued Jesus and touched His hem because she knew who He was.* Because she was obedient to what was in her spirit, she acted immediately. That is undeniable faith. Elder Desirie once said, "so many people were touching Jesus in the huge crowd, and out of everyone there, He felt her touch His hem, because of her great faith it caused Jesus to stop."

She defied all things in the natural to access that in the spiritual and did what she knew would change her whole life. It was not a whiny, begging, sniveling, fearful, soulish faith, but a determined, absolutely-nothing-could-stop-her, kind of revelation faith. She defied the possibility of being stoned to death because she knew He was the Savior, and He would give her life. So, I asked myself, what will I defy, deny, and defeat in my own life to go after God . . . Everything!

Meditation Scriptures

Romans 10:17 WNT

And this proves that faith comes from a Message heard, and that the Message comes through its having been *spoken* by Christ.

Mark 4:24 NLT

Then he added, "Pay close attention to what you hear. The closer you listen, the more understanding you will be given—and you will receive even more.

Proverbs 3:5-6 ESV

Trust in the Lord with all your heart, and do not lean on your own understanding. In all your ways acknowledge him, and he will make straight your paths.

2 Corinthians 5:7 ESV

For we walk by faith, not by sight.

John 15:7 AMP

If you remain in Me and My words remain in you [that is, if we are vitally united and My message lives in your heart], ask whatever you wish and it will be done for you.

Psalms 36:6-11 CJB

Adonai, in the heavens is your grace; your faithfulness reaches to the skies. Your righteousness is like the mountains of God, your judgments are like the great deep. You save man and beast, *Adonai*.

How precious, God, is your grace! People take refuge in the shadow of your wings, they feast on the rich bounty of your house, and you have them drink from the stream of your delights. For with you is the fountain of life; in your light we see light. Continue your grace to those who know you and your righteousness to the upright in heart.

Psalm 115:14-16 NLT

May the Lord richly bless both you and your children. *May you be blessed by the Lord,* who made heaven and earth. The heavens belong to the Lord, but he has given the earth to all humanity.

CHAPTER 18:
THE FIRE, THE BATTLEGROUND, THE TESTING

"They will be like mighty warriors in battle, trampling their enemies in the mud under their feet. Since the Lord is with them as they fight, they will overthrow even the enemy's horsemen."

(Zechariah 10:5 NLT)

"Now this is what the LORD says—He who created you, O Jacob, and He who formed you, O Israel: "Do not fear, for I have redeemed you; I have called you by your name; you are Mine! When you pass through the waters, I will be with you; and when you go through the rivers, they will not overwhelm you. When you walk through the fire, you will not be scorched; the flames will not set you ablaze."

(Isaiah 43:1-2 BSB)

When I first walked back into the church in 2015, I would cringe every time someone was teaching about being tested or going through a battle. There was nothing I detested more than adversity and the fire. By this time, I had been going through so many things for 15 years. So many years lost. I just remember thinking, "these people don't even know what a battle really is." But they did, their battles were just different than mine!

Many times, I was so unprepared for any kind of testing or battle for so many years—praying out of tears, begging, and desperation, not really knowing the Word of God or the voice of God. I was taught and believed that memorizing scripture and reciting verses was enough, even though it rarely yielded any fruit, I never desired to go beyond this. We often do what we are taught religiously without question, believing that we are all to do the same thing to get the same results, but that is not living faith.

When the enemy attacks, it is a step by step process many times. Marriages that are great do not suddenly end one morning; so many smaller battles must be lost before that happens. The devil has a precise plan of attack to destroy an area in our lives, and we often don't see what is happening until much has been destroyed. I was so oblivious to the tactics of the enemy that I put up no resistance until I had lost way too much.

It was often as though I was fighting the enemy blindfolded using inadequate weapons or weapons that I did not know how to use. I would swing aimlessly in the dark hoping to hit something, but the enemy always had the upper hand. Without knowing what to expect, or the enemies plans, or which weapons to use, I was unprepared for each battle. Without adequate training, I could not take up the weapons of my warfare and use them effectively.

THE FIRE, THE BATTLE GROUND THE TESTING

I walked fearfully into battle after battle with my victory already relinquished to the enemy and wondered why I could not come out victorious. Trying to walk into battle with someone else's armor or a generic battle plan will not work. Out of fear, I always anticipated another attack but was still surprised when these attacks hit, and I just stood there in shock or tears. I would take all the hits from the enemy until I could stand it no longer and then cry out to God. Then I would try to start fighting with very little strength or wisdom. I accepted my defeats as God's will or made excuses for why something did not turn out right, when God was wanting so much more for me.

I had more faith in the fire itself than I did in God. God is always preparing us, not just through the Bible, but through His Spirit. Reading and studying is only the first step and is vital, but God wants us to go much further than this. When He is requiring more of you, you will not walk in faith until you are obedient.

I rarely dream of anything at all, but when I do, I pay attention to every detail. At the beginning of 2019, I had a dream where my home was attacked by homeless people. They were outside at first, parked in front of my house, pretending to have car trouble in a beat up old, rusted station wagon. They rushed toward me as I was entering my home, and as they walked in, their true identity was revealed.

They were witches assigned to me in ugly black clothing. These demons had singled me out and invaded my home quickly. So, I hid my kids and grandkids, and locked them away safely, but left myself vulnerable to their attacks. I do not remember whether they had weapons or not, but I feared for our lives. They were ransacking my home, taking what they wanted. At first, there were three of them, but I began to see them multiply in numbers right before my eyes. I wanted them gone, so I was negotiating with them, telling them I would give them all my food and all my money if they just left. They took what I offered and continued to multiply and take even more.

When I woke up, I was so upset because I had totally been unarmed and unprepared for this attack, but most of all I was upset because I was alone. I did not know where Mario was. I knew I was defenseless by myself. There is no negotiating with the devil. I had to be armed, ready and on the offense. But most of all we had to be unified. No longer would I leave myself susceptible to the attacks of the enemy. I had to double check all my defenses. I could not walk blindly without faith and wait to be attacked again.

As I readied myself for battle, I realized the fire, or the battleground, is an amazing place if you let God do what He has destined for you. When we walk into a storm, our first inclination is to run, but that is the worst thing you can do. These are times where God wants to lead, protect, surround, and enable us. It is where you can watch God fight for you and defend you. It's where miracles can happen. It is when you are surrounded by the enemy that God shows up in power and strength. It's where lives are changed.

We pray for God to take us out of the fire when that is the best place to be. That is where His love is so evident and fierce. That is where, if you are focused on God, His presence is so overwhelming. It is where the true peace of God is manifested and profound. That is where you are purified of the old nature, and His life is revealed through you, bringing such amazing freedom. Those things that are not of God are burned away. But what happens after the fire, after the victory, is even more amazing! I will talk about that later . . .

Isaiah 59:19 KJV

So shall they fear the name of the Lord from the west, and his glory from the rising of the sun. When the enemy shall come in like a flood, the Spirit of the Lord shall lift up a standard against him.

1 Peter 1:6-7 BSB

In this you greatly rejoice, though now for a little while you may have had to suffer grief in various trials so that the proven character of your faith— more precious than gold, which perishes even though refined by fire— may result in praise, glory, and honor at the revelation of Jesus Christ.

The fire may be uncomfortable, it may be hard at times, things will be required of us and sacrifices must be made, but the outcome will bring new life. The fire reveals who you are and exposes those things that are not pleasing to God—the junk in our life. Just as in the natural, a forest fire clears the way of debris, it also nourishes the soil, releases new seeds, and allows life to spring forth when the rain begins to fall. It purges the dead and clears a way for new life.

When we go through the fire, it is not only to purify us of those unholy things in our lives, but it also burns away the enemies that defile us. It destroys so many strongholds. Those things that we could not get rid of on our own cannot withstand the fire. When I walked out of the fire, I was so much more alive than I had ever been, and my spiritual clarity was so intense. So much weight on my shoulders instantly disappeared!

We don't have to go through the difficult times barely making it through. Many times, in the past 20 years, it felt like I crawled out of the dark valley, bloody and broken. I would barely come up for air when I would be dragged back in again. I came out of many fires alive, but badly burned. This is not victory. *Surviving is not victory.* Tears do not mean you have been changed or delivered. When I looked at the outcome of these battles, I did not see any type of victory or positive change in me. I came out in worse shape than before. Not anymore. I never say I am a "Breast Cancer Survivor" because I did not just survive. I have triumphed over and came out victorious because of Almighty God. And I will never speak any other name over my life again.

When we are truly hidden away in God, the storms will not even phase us. We can go through the fire never feeling the heat. Surviving does not bring God nearly as much glory as walking through victorious.

One powerful passage God had me study was regarding Shadrach, Meshach, and Abednego. When they were put in the fire, they already knew who God was, the extent of their faith exceeded anything they saw in the natural. Never did they concern themselves with the situation, the outcome, or the fire, but only in their God. They were not going to bow to anyone else but Yahweh, and their faith infuriated the enemy.

They went in bound but came out free! The only thing that got burned in the fire was what the enemy tried to bind them with, and the enemy's strongest soldiers!!! These believers did not crawl out of the furnace smelling

THE FIRE, THE BATTLE GROUND THE TESTING

like smoke or blackened by ash. They did not just make it out of the fire barely alive, they prospered. This was a true test of their faith, and it was dependent on their unwillingness to compromise. Don't fear in the fire!

If their relationship with God was superficial or religious, they would not have survived. If they had huddled together and quoted scripture that they did not have a revelation on, they would have died. If they did not know God for who He is, they would have burned. They knew way before they walked into the furnace that God was able!

Jesus was present in that fire for the whole world to see why they were victorious. He did not remove them from the ordeal, but took them through the fire unharmed and victorious! That is true faith. But it didn't stop there. Their enemy now believed in their God and favored these men! And those who saw the fourth man in the fire, feared this God, the one that Shadrach, Meshach and Abednego served!

If you saw what was on the other side of the battle, and what was to come after victory, you would never give up. If you understood who else will be changed by your victory, you would run to the fire. You would be willing to be obedient for the sake of your loved ones. Our sight must go beyond the giants before us, beyond the fire we are stepping into. When it is all over, and you have victory, you will question why you ever wavered, why you ever feared. *After the battle, after the victory, there is so much more!*

The devil thought he was going to put me in the furnace bound again, but I went in free and came out free! He thought I would give up, but instead my faith enraged him. He thought I would die in the fire alone, but I came out more alive than ever, I was never alone, and I knew it all along. Jesus walked with me through this last surgery so people could see who God is! So God could be glorified. There is no mistaking who was with me and what He did for me!

THE FIRE, THE BATTLE GROUND THE TESTING

Meditation Scriptures

Ephesians 6:14-20 AMP

So stand firm *and* hold your ground, having tightened the wide band of truth (personal integrity, moral courage) around your waist and having put on the breastplate of righteousness (an upright heart), and having strapped on your feet the gospel of peace in preparation [to face the enemy with firm-footed stability and the readiness produced by the good news]. Above all, lift up the [protective] shield of faith with which you can extinguish all the flaming arrows of the evil *one*. And take the helmet of salvation, and the sword of the Spirit, which is the Word of God.

With all prayer and petition pray *[with specific requests]* at all times [on every occasion and in every season] in the Spirit, and with this in view, stay alert with all perseverance and petition [interceding in prayer] for all God's people. And *pray* for me, that words may be given to me when I open my mouth, to proclaim boldly the mystery of the good news [of salvation], for which I am an ambassador in chains. And *pray* that in *proclaiming* it I may speak boldly *and* courageously, as I should.

Psalm 84:5-7 AMP

Blessed *and* greatly favored is the man whose strength is in You, In whose heart are the highways *to Zion*.
Passing through the Valley of Weeping, they make it a place of springs; The early rain also covers it with blessings. They go from strength to strength [increasing in victorious power];
Each of them appears before God in Zion.

Daniel 3:16-28 NLT

Shadrach, Meshach, and Abednego replied, "O Nebuchadnezzar, we do not need to defend ourselves before you. If we are thrown into the blazing furnace, the God whom we serve is able to save us. He will rescue us from your power, Your Majesty. But even if he doesn't, we want to make it clear to you, Your Majesty, that we will never serve your gods or worship the gold statue you have set up."

Nebuchadnezzar was so furious with Shadrach, Meshach, and Abednego that his face became distorted with rage. He commanded that the furnace be heated seven times hotter than usual. Then he ordered some of the strongest men of his army to bind Shadrach, Meshach, and Abednego and throw them into the blazing furnace. So they tied them up and threw them into the furnace, fully dressed in their pants, turbans, robes, and other garments. And because the king, in his anger, had demanded such a hot fire in the furnace, the flames killed the soldiers as they threw the three men in. So Shadrach, Meshach, and Abednego, securely tied, fell into the roaring flames. But suddenly, Nebuchadnezzar jumped up in amazement and exclaimed to his advisers, "Didn't we tie up three men and throw them into the furnace?" "Yes, Your Majesty, we certainly did," they replied. "Look!" Nebuchadnezzar shouted. "I see four men, unbound, walking around in the fire unharmed! And the fourth looks like a god!" Then Nebuchadnezzar came as close as he could to the door of the flaming furnace and shouted: "Shadrach, Meshach, and Abednego, servants of the Most High God, come out! Come here!" So Shadrach, Meshach, and Abednego stepped out of the fire. Then the high officers, officials, governors, and advisers crowded around them and saw that the fire had not touched them. Not a hair on their heads was singed, and their clothing was not scorched. They didn't even smell of smoke!

Then Nebuchadnezzar said, "Praise to the God of Shadrach, Meshach, and Abednego! He sent his angel to rescue his servants who trusted in him. They defied the king's command and were willing to die rather than serve or worship any god except their own God. Therefore, I make this decree: If any people, whatever their race or nation or language, speak a word against the God of Shadrach, Meshach, and Abednego, they will be torn limb from limb, and their houses will be turned into heaps of rubble. There is no other god who can rescue like this!" Then the king promoted Shadrach, Meshach, and Abednego to even higher positions in the province of Babylon.

CHAPTER 19:
OBEDIENCE

"If we [claim to] live by the [Holy] Spirit, we must also walk by the Spirit [with personal integrity, godly character, and moral courage—our conduct empowered by the Holy Spirit]."

(Galatians 5:25 AMP)

"And this is love: that we walk in obedience to his commands. As you have heard from the beginning, his command is that you walk in love."

(2 John 1:6)

Years of living the effects of all my unruliness opened my eyes to one basic action to faith: Obedience. I was doing the opposite of what God wanted in everything, and I was reaping the results. Pure and simple, faith is following God's voice in everything, and I mean everything. Not the pastor's voice, not your best friend's voice, not the voice preaching on the internet, not your own voice. Obedience only comes with relationship, and relationship only comes through surrender.

Out of love for God and trust, I wanted to be obedient. Because of this desire, He showed me who He was and continues to show me more each day. The freedom that comes from surrendering to Him is unlike anything else you will ever experience. In dying you will live! We have only experienced a minuscule amount of the life He wants to give us. There is so much more.

The whole year prior to this last surgery, He led me on a path that I could not always grasp at the time, but I never questioned it. Sometimes, it seemed like it did not make any sense, or like I was going in circles, but it was all precise steps down a path where I was fully dependent on Him, where I came alive in Christ. The more I submitted, the more I heard His voice; the easier it got to be obedient, the more I fell in love with Him.

There is such a liberating freedom in unquestionable obedience. He was ordering my every step. He taught me great and mighty things. He hid me away. He ravished me with himself. I never asked for material blessing but only more of Him. And He was faithful to that request every single time.

With this last surgery I had no alternate plan, what I would do if everything turned out bad. There were no longer thoughts of how I would survive this surgery if things went wrong, I had for 20 years always imagined the worst, anxiously awaited the next bad thing to happen, and mentally prepared for the next big disaster. That is not faith. Living like this for 20 years was torment. But not this time! All I cared about now was the presence of God.

There was no mental preparation for the surgery like I had tried to do so many times before, because that is not of God. That is not faith. I didn't need to prepare my emotions, I needed to reinforce my strong tower. I needed to be hidden away. I needed to know my God! That's exactly what I did. There was only preparation for the battle through the Spirit of God. All I needed to do was jump in that river and rest in what God wanted to do in me. Because I did not concern myself with my mind or my emotions, but only my spirit, they had no authority over me. *Who or what (God or your emotions) you give your attention to and pursue, will have victory over your life.*

When I went into this surgery, I was completely confident in my God because I truly knew Him by what He wanted me to know this year. I had finally entered into the rest of faith, knowing full well that God was in control. This victory was *already* a tangible manifestation of God's love for me. Everything that He showed me about himself, I wanted more of. I saw exactly what He wanted me to see in Him, forgetting all that I already knew and starting from scratch.

Each characteristic of God became alive to me as I searched Him out in that specific area. If He told me to search out His love, the deeper I went; the more He could manifest that characteristic to me, the more I wanted. Initially, it was a little hard because I was so unsure of His voice, but soon it was all so easy, and then it became crucial, my deepest desire. It all started because of obedience to his voice, obedience to one small but powerful command, *"Just worship me."*

Meditation Scriptures

Romans 8:14 AMP

For all who are *allowing themselves to* be led by the Spirit of God are sons of God.

Psalm 119:130 AMPC

The entrance *and* unfolding of Your words give light; their unfolding gives understanding (discernment and comprehension) to the simple.

Luke 11:28 NIV

He replied, "Blessed rather are those who hear the word of God and obey it."

2 Timothy 3:16-17 ESV

All Scripture is breathed out by God and profitable for teaching, for reproof, for correction, and for training in righteousness, that the man of God may be complete, equipped for every good work.

Colossians 3:1-2 BSB

Therefore, since you have been raised with Christ, strive for the things above, where Christ is seated at the right hand of God. Set your minds on things above, not on earthly things. For you died, and your life is now hidden with Christ in God.

Psalm 57:1

Be merciful to me, O God, be merciful to me, for in you my soul takes refuge; in the shadow of your wings I will take refuge, till the storms of destruction pass by.

OBEDIENCE

Hebrews 3:19 AMPC

So we see that they were not able to enter [into His rest], because of their unwillingness to adhere to *and* trust in *and* rely on God [unbelief had shut them out].

1 Corinthians 2:4-16 NLT

Yet when I am among mature believers, I do speak with words of wisdom, but not the kind of wisdom that belongs to this world or to the rulers of this world, who are soon *forgotten.* No, the wisdom we speak of is the mystery of God—his plan that was previously hidden, even though He made it for our ultimate glory before the world began. But the rulers of this world have not understood it; if they had, they would not have crucified our glorious Lord. That is what the Scriptures mean when they say, "*No eye has seen, no ear has heard, and no mind has imagined what God has prepared for those who love him.*" But it was to us that God revealed these things by his Spirit. *For his Spirit searches out everything and shows us God's deep secrets.* No one can know a person's thoughts except that person's own spirit, and no one can know God's thoughts except God's own Spirit. And we have received God's Spirit (not the world's spirit), so we can know the wonderful things God has freely given us. When we tell you these things, we do not use words that come from human wisdom. Instead, *we speak words given to us by the Spirit,* using the Spirit's words to explain spiritual truths. But people who aren't spiritual can't receive these truths from God's Spirit. It all sounds foolish to them and they can't understand it, for only those who are spiritual can understand what the Spirit means. Those who are spiritual can evaluate all things, but they themselves cannot be evaluated by others. For, "Who can know the Lord's thoughts? Who knows enough to teach him?"

CHAPTER 20: VICTORY

"For every child of God defeats this evil world, and we achieve this victory through our faith. And who can win this battle against the world? Only those who believe that Jesus is the Son of God."

(1 John 5:4-5 NLT)

Late 2018, and as I went into 2019, I knew God was speaking strongly to me about *victory*. That was the word He gave me for this year, and it kept coming up in my spirit all year. As I began to walk down this path, with each step, I wanted more and more of God, so I followed Him wherever He went. I would study about victory often, and read everything I could about the battles, the enemies, and the victories, as well as the defeats, but mostly about the love of God that surrounded His people in these victories. These battles became alive, and God spoke to me often about them.

Throughout the year, God would speak specific words and scriptures to me that I did not know or study, and I knew that that was what I had to proclaim, meditate on, and search out. When I spoke these words, there was power behind them. When I quoted the scripture He would bring forth in my spirit, things would begin to manifest. It was a puzzle that He was showing me one piece at a time, but at that time, I still did not have the full picture. I did not know why.

Galatians 3:5-7 ESV

Does he who supplies the Spirit to you and works miracles among you do so by works of the law, or <u>by hearing with faith</u>?

Journal Entry 12/20/2018

The rock that slew the giant is God's living word (rhema) He gives us for that situation. Victory is my word for this year 2019. This word I will proclaim everyday. His word cannot fail because my victory will bring victory to all Israel. Many will witness His victory in my life. And I will proclaim victory for others. They shall see the Lord move on their behalf and give Him glory!

This entry was exactly one year before the actual day of my final surgery! I had no idea when I was going to have the final surgery or if I would ever do it. I had not remembered what I wrote, or even understood it fully, until recently while preparing to write this book over a year later. This was just the beginning of everything He wanted to teach me for the next year, but I had to proclaim this first. I had to believe His voice. This was God showing me clearly what was to come. Because of obedience, I watched as that giant fell to the ground!

OBEDIENCE

Exodus 15:1-3, 7, 12, 13 (NLT)

Then Moses and the people of Israel sang this song to the Lord: "I will sing to the Lord, for he has triumphed gloriously; he has hurled both horse and rider into the sea. The Lord is my strength and my song; he has given me victory. This is my God, and I will praise him—my father's God, and I will exalt him!

The Lord is a warrior; Yahweh is his name! "Your right hand, O Lord, is glorious in power.

Your right hand, O Lord, smashes the enemy. In the greatness of your majesty, you overthrow those who rise against you. You unleash your blazing fury; it consumes them like straw. "Who is like you among the gods, O Lord—glorious in holiness, awesome in splendor, performing great wonders? You raised your right hand,

and the earth swallowed our enemies. "With your unfailing love you lead the people you have redeemed.
In your might, you guide them to your sacred home.

Victory is not the outcome of your battle. It is not the belief that you will have victory if you go through the battle. It comes way before the end of the fight or even the beginning of an attack. Victory does not come when you don't know the Conqueror, the Victor: Jesus. You cannot have victory when you don't know what victory is. You can never have victory in the flesh. I tried that for so long. Victory does not come from desperation. God in His mercy will be faithful to His word, but we make it so much harder than it has to be. Sometimes, we get victory in a situation, but we don't know why it happens. We think God just suddenly decides to bless us and take us out of a situation.

There were many times over my life when I knew God intervened and His mercy overtook me. But I needed to understand why so many times I was not walking in victory and authority. I had to understand how to live in victory and bring victory to others. I wanted and sought after revelation on victory, healings, fire, trials, and tests, but most of all I wanted revelation of God himself.

Your victory is not in the outcome. It's a journey where you must walk with God in victory. The outcome is already in God's hands, it is His heart. I had victory this time because I walked in it before this ever happened, and because I walked in the evidence He gave me which was His spoken word. Preparation for battle is knowing you have the victory. It is seeking our Victor, the one who triumphed over death.

Luke 14:31 ESV

Or what king, going out to encounter another king in war, will not sit down first and deliberate whether he is able with ten thousand to meet him who comes against him with twenty thousand?

Sometimes, we want to proclaim victory halfway through the fight, but without going into the battle confident of who God is, it will be an uphill battle. When God sent armies to fight, they went in led by the voice of God, knowing they would be victorious when they walked in obedience. When they were not obedient, they were defeated. How many armies go to war if they are not sure they can win or do not have a battle plan? They are trained, motivated, and assured they will win. They go to battle prepared. Not a general preparation but specific to that enemy.

OBEDIENCE

Joshua 10:8 NLT

"Do not be afraid of them," the Lord said to Joshua, "<u>for I have given you victory</u> over them. Not a single one of them will be able to stand up to you."

Those battles I went through for 20 years, when not walking in the perfect plan of God, when not surrounded by God, brought fear, defeat, trauma, panic, and bitterness. I came out far more injured than when I went in. God does not want us barely surviving. He secured the victory and yet we walk in defeat. I went kicking and screaming into each fight but this last one I looked forward to. This time I was ready. Not once did I question where He was or even how He was going to take care of me through this. I already knew.

So many live in defeat for years, like my Apostle Kem says, "Broke, busted, and disgusted," needlessly, when all has been sacrificed for us. If we do no not have victory, it is because we do not know God, we do not desire God, and we do not pursue God. If we did, then hearing His voice and obedience would be easy, second nature, and victory would be spontaneous.

He does not want us to be tormented while we are going through the battle. We do not even have to be affected by what's going on around us. We can walk in victory continuously, not randomly. We can command with absolute authority the outcome of a situation without fear, and we can be prepared for any attacks way before they come. It only comes through relationship, and only through surrendered obedience to his voice.

Daniel 2:22 AMPC

He reveals the deep and secret things; He knows what is in the darkness, and the light dwells with Him!

Zechariah 13:9 NABRE

I will bring the one third through the fire; I will refine them as one refines silver, and I will test them as one tests gold. They will call upon my name, and I will answer them; I will say, "They are my people," and they will say, "The Lord is my God."

Victory is you walking out God's perfect will, through obedience, and when the enemy is not only defeated but justice is served. Victory is knowing who God is. Victory is the absence of fear because you have a revelation of God's love. Victory is his spoken word to you. I saw this all before I was in the operating room. It was not a question of waiting to see a manifestation of His promises or when it might happen. I already saw that it was manifested in my spirit! I was already walking as though it was guaranteed and rejoicing in the victory I knew was mine.

It is only by being led by His Spirit in prayer, study, and abiding with God are we able to allow God to fight our battles and hand us the victory. God watches over His Word to make sure it does what it is destined to do. But first He reveals it to us so that we can align our faith to His exact will in every situation.

OBEDIENCE

John 4:23-24 TPT

From here on, worshiping the Father will not be a matter of the right place but with the right heart. For God is a Spirit, and he longs to have sincere worshipers who worship and adore him in the realm of the Spirit and in truth."

In order to live victoriously, you must also realize what worship really is: full access for God to do what is necessary in our lives, a stance of victory, and most of all, an intimacy with the one that loves us so intently and completely. Worship opens our hearts and cultivates our ground to become a place where the seed of the Word of God can flourish. Worship brings the rain of God to our spirits! Worship brings clarity to His voice in us as He expresses His heart for us.

When we declare who God is in worship, and what He has said to our spirits, we give Him full authority to act on our behalf, we claim our rights, we declare who we belong to, we bring into manifestation our faith; and we announce with joy who our victor is! The enemy is brutally reminded that we are guaranteed the victory, and we will not relinquish our promises, leaving him confused and powerless. But being a worshipper must be your lifeline, part of who you are naturally, a deep desire that starts way before any battle is eminent.

Psalms 5:7-8 NLT

Because of your unfailing love, I can enter your house; I will worship at your Temple with deepest awe.
Lead me in the right path, O Lord, or my enemies will conquer me. Make your way plain for me to follow.

After all the trauma I went through for years, it was becoming so evident and so surreal to me the high price Jesus paid. I suffered greatly in ways I never expected, but He experienced so much for me and for every person who ever existed. He paid a price too great to bear except through the power of God. This is why I worship Him and Him alone. I do not take God for granted, knowing all that He has done for me.

You will never see me complacent during worship because I know who I serve now. I know the level of my victory will be determined by the depth of my worship. I can no longer contain the greatness of the God inside of me! My life is his sanctuary, and my voice is His battle cry!

Worship deepens your desire for even more of God. Worship causes you to trust God when the darkness surrounds you. Victory comes from knowing God will never leave your side, and it comes from wanting God more than anything else.

Psalm 29:2 TPT

Be in awe before his majesty. Be in awe before such power and might! Come worship wonderful Yahweh, arrayed in all his splendor, bowing in worship as he appears in the beauty of holiness.

Give him the honor due his name. Worship him wearing the glory-garments of your holy, priestly calling!

OBEDIENCE

Psalm 107:14-16 TPT

His light broke through the darkness and he led us out in freedom from death's dark shadow and snapped every one of our chains. **So lift your hands and give thanks to God for his marvelous kindness** *and for his miracles of mercy for those he loves!* **For he smashed through heavy prison doors and** *shattered the steel bars that held us back, just to set us free!*

Psalm 59:16 TPT

But as for me, your strength shall be my song of joy. At each and every sunrise, my lyrics of your love will fill the air! For you have been my glory-fortress, a stronghold in my day of distress.

Journal Entry 12/17/19

3 nights before my final surgery

I was already in the future looking back at this victory like it already happened.

This time, I walked in victory into the battle. This time, I walked into the battle in the spirit. This time, I knew who God was, and His love for me could not let me be defeated. Victory was mine before the battle started, even before the mental battle started. Why? Because I took that victory and made it mine. I sought God and He led me into understanding His love, His faithfulness, His greatness, His authority, and my authority. The victory that was guaranteed to me, signed for by the blood of Jesus. A victory that includes recompense and justice. I have triumphed over fear and death and rejoiced before the battle began. I studied the enemy, the battle plan God designed just *for me, the attributes of a warrior, and most of all, the faithfulness and goodness of God. I had to know beyond words who God is. I had to know who I am. I had to allow God to plant this faith inside of me, by Him impregnating me with words He had predestined before I was created. To grow my faith by revelation, I had to allow those words to grow within me. I had to bring them to term and deliver them and let them live and thrive. I had to be obedient to God's spoken Word to me in each season.*

Psalms 42:7 NIV

Deep calls to deep in the roar of your waterfalls; all your waves and breakers have swept over me.

1 John 4:4 NLT

But you belong to God, my dear children. <u>You have already won a victory</u> over those people, because the Spirit who lives in you is greater than the spirit who lives in the world.

I had the victory before the battle. I saw this battle through a victorious heart because that was my harvest from what God had planted in me through the seeds of faith by His spoken Word into my spirit. He cultivated this victory when I sought after him. He provided rain for these seeds of victory each time I went into worship.He provided this victory because of His faithfulness, because of His love, and because He cannot be defeated. That is who He is to me.

There was no way that God would be unfaithful to me or to what He planted in me, and I was more sure of this than anything. These statements are not emotions or knowledge, but so true to my heart that no one can ever convince me otherwise. They are part of me now, and their roots are deep. There was no way I could be defeated because there was no way God could be defeated, and He is in me, with me, and for me. He cannot deny himself, nor can He deny *everything he spoke to me,* because it was alive and producing a harvest of victory.

God gave me much more than a plan of attack, I had a guarantee that I already won. It was not a struggle. Fear did not have a chokehold on me. I was never desperate. Before I got to that day of the surgery, I had done all that was required of me; I proclaimed the scriptures God told me that were specifically for me, I studied who He is by his Spirit, I understood what victory is, and I went into prayer time, and time and time again, followed His lead every step of the way. When I did this, I was consumed by Him, overshadowed by Him. It was His master plan. I had finally known what being hidden away in God really is.

When it came time for the battle, I literally sat still in the presence of God and watched Him fight for me. But not only for me, but also for my children and my grandchildren for a thousand generations! You cannot do that when you have barely made it out of the last battle and are still fighting with your own battle plan and not God's battle plan.

Surviving a battle does not mean you have the victory. Living through the fire does not mean it changed you for the better. I survived battle after battle but had no victory until now. It was always God having mercy on me, which was great, but I needed to stand in this battle and take authority by His

Spirit. I had to learn what authority was and that it only comes through relationship and obedience.

Even though I already triumphed over this, I had to still go through the surgery so that the glory of God could be manifested and acknowledged in my life. So that in this victory, it could be evident to others what is vital. And so that all that He taught me could not be disputed.

Now, I could tell my testimony because now it would bring glory to God. Now, I saw how it all worked together. Now, I was walking in my true inheritance. Now, I walked in victory that was very costly to my life, but so worth every tear and every ounce of pain. Now, my testimony is a worship unto God, a triumphant praise, a thunderous roar to Almighty God, chasing enemies far away. Now, I cannot settle for anything less than being triumphant in everything. Now, I will not let my brother or sister walk alone down that same desolate road I traveled for so long. Whatever you have been victorious through creates a bridge for others to cross over!

OBEDIENCE

Meditation Scriptures

2 Chronicles 20:17 NLT

But *you will not even need to fight. Take your positions; then stand still and watch the Lord's victory.* He is with you, O people of Judah and Jerusalem. Do not be afraid or discouraged. Go out against them tomorrow, for the Lord is with you!"

Psalm 27 AMP
The Lord is my light and my salvation—
Whom shall I fear?
The Lord is the refuge and fortress of my life—
Whom shall I dread?
When the wicked came against me to eat up my flesh,
My adversaries and my enemies, they stumbled and fell.
Though an army encamp against me,
My heart will not fear;
Though war arise against me,
Even in this I am confident.
One thing I have asked of the Lord, and that I will seek:
That I may dwell in the house of the Lord [in His presence] all the days of my life,
To gaze upon the beauty [the delightful loveliness and majestic grandeur] of the Lord
And to meditate in His temple.
For in the day of trouble He will hide me in His shelter;
In the secret place of His tent He will hide me;
He will lift me up on a rock.
And now my head will be lifted up above my enemies around me,
In His tent I will offer sacrifices with shouts of joy;
I will sing, yes, I will sing praises to the Lord.

Hear, O Lord, when I cry aloud;
Be gracious and compassionate to me and answer me.
When You said, "Seek My face [in prayer, require My presence as your greatest need]," my heart said to You,
"Your face, O Lord, I will seek [on the authority of Your word]."
Do not hide Your face from me,
Do not turn Your servant away in anger;
You have been my help;
Do not abandon me nor [a]leave me,
O God of my salvation!
Although my father and my mother have abandoned me,
Yet the Lord will take me up [adopt me as His child].
Teach me Your way, O Lord,
And lead me on a level path
Because of my enemies [who lie in wait].
Do not give me up to the will of my adversaries,
For false witnesses have come against me;
They breathe out violence.
I would have despaired had I not believed that I would see the goodness of the Lord
In the land of the living.
Wait for and confidently expect the Lord;
Be strong and let your heart take courage;
Yes, wait for and confidently expect the Lord.

Psalm 138:3 AMP
On the day I called, You answered me;
And You made me bold and confident with [renewed] strength in my life.

OBEDIENCE

Exodus 15:1-3 NLT

Then Moses and the people of Israel sang this song to the Lord: "I will sing to the Lord, for he has triumphed gloriously; he has hurled both horse and rider into the sea. The Lord is my strength and my song; he has given me victory. This is my God, and I will praise him—my father's God, and I will exalt him!
The Lord is a warrior; Yahweh is his name!

Romans 8:16-17 MSG

This resurrection life you received from God is not a timid, grave-tending life. It's adventurously expectant, greeting God with a childlike "What's next, Papa?" God's Spirit touches our spirits and confirms who we really are. We know who he is, and we know who we are: Father and children. And we know we are going to get what's coming to us—an unbelievable inheritance! We go through exactly what Christ goes through. If we go through the hard times with him, then we're certainly going to go through the good times with him!

1 Peter 2:9 NLT

But you are not like that, for you are a chosen people. You are royal priests, a holy nation, God's very own possession. As a result, you can show others the goodness of God, for he called you out of the darkness into his wonderful light.

John 14:26-27 NLT

But when the Father sends the Advocate as my representative—that is, the Holy Spirit—he will teach you everything and will remind you of everything I have told you.

"I am leaving you with a gift—peace of mind and heart. And the peace I give is a gift the world cannot give. So don't be troubled or afraid.

CHAPTER 21:
OUR JOB

"Call to Me, and I will answer you, and show you great and mighty things, which you do not know."

(Jeremiah 33:30 NKJV)

"Let me hear Your lovingkindness in the morning, For I trust in You. Teach me the way in which I should walk, For I lift up my soul to You."

(Psalms 143:8 AMP)

An intimate relationship with God can't be obtained on Sundays alone. It cannot even be obtained by daily devotionals, memorizing scripture, just reading the Bible, and rehearsing prayers. It will not be obtained by church BBQs, fellowships, conferences, or Bible studies. I thought for so long because I gave of my money and time that I had a relationship with God. But during every battle, I was lost. I wanted God to show up on my timing, for my need and in my way. My life was about me and because of that, I almost lost everything.

God wants to show you the most effective path, and the weapons of your warfare, but most of all, He wants your heart. Not just when you are born-again and going to church, not just in your prayer closet, or when you have an urgent need; and not just learning from the pulpit and reading the word. He wants to give life to the Word, speak to you through it in your spirit, and show you who He really is. Without the Holy Spirit, our helper guiding us in every step, we are doing it in our own strength!!!

Romans 12:1-2 BSB

Therefore I urge you, brothers, on account of God's mercy, to offer your bodies as living sacrifices, holy and pleasing to God, which is your spiritual service of worship. Do not be conformed to this world, but be transformed by the <u>renewing of your mind. Then you will be able to test and approve what is the good, pleasing, and perfect will of God</u>

Read and pray and study and worship, but when God tells you to go on a specific path, be obedient, because that is where your anointing lies. That is where the power to slay the giant lies. That is where God's truths are incisive. Have trust in the voice of God within you to direct your path. Build your confidence in His voice, learn to trust even the small things that He says because they will be life to you, and they are true to your life. Do not rely only on what you are being taught. There were so many times when after a preaching at church, God showed me so much more, He expanded it and illuminated what was taught—but only when I searched Him out in everything. Sometimes, God even gave me the message before it was preached by our pastor.

OUR JOB

Proverbs 8:17 AMPC

I love those who love me, and those who seek me early and diligently shall find me.

You will never be disappointed when you lay down everything and search for the hidden things of God. Find that secret place that God has just for you, where He can show you who He is and surround you with peace. It is where nothing else in the world will matter because you will know you are loved by God Almighty! For me, this was my special beach in La Jolla, which was like my "Garden of Gethsemane and Garden of Eden." Where I enjoyed the abundance of His presence, where I poured out my heart and tears to God, where I surrendered my will, and where God gave me the assurance that I had victory.

1 Chronicles 16:11 AMPC

Seek the Lord and His strength; yearn for and seek His face and to be in His presence continually!

Do not underestimate what God has put inside of you and what He wants to do for you. It is more than you think! He is willing to take you as deep as you want to go! Being obedient to his Spirit is the next step to intimacy, this is where the glory is obtained. So seek after that level of oneness where his voice leads you through the path of the Word of God and through your life, where your weapons are those things that you know deep down in your heart that no enemy can withstand.

Even in hearing His voice and instructions, God's perfect timing is essential. He may give you prophecies for years, like He did me about the gift of miracles and healings. But I could not walk in that or even pursue those gifts, until it was the appointed time. He is always telling us what is to come to give us faith. And He is always, always, always preparing things for the promises He has given us. It may seem like an endless amount of time, but when you walk in it, time becomes nothing. The wait is insignificant when compared to the blessings of walking in His perfect will. The longer the journey, the sweeter the victory, and the journey is just as important as the destination!

CHAPTER 22:
MY ROCK

"Your lovingkindness and graciousness, O Lord, extend to the skies, Your faithfulness [reaches] to the clouds. Your righteousness is like the mountains of God, Your judgments are like the great deep ocean. O Lord, You preserve man and beast. How precious is Your lovingkindness, O God!

The children of men take refuge in the shadow of Your wings. They drink their fill of the abundance of Your house; And You allow them to drink from the river of Your delights. For with You is the fountain of life [the fountain of life-giving water]; In Your light we see light. O continue Your lovingkindness to those who know You, And Your righteousness (salvation) to the upright in heart."

(Psalm 36:5-10 AMP)

When I went for my post ops, a few weeks after my surgery, I stopped by our beach to walk and talk with God. Thankfulness and joy were overflowing from my heart as I walked out onto the silky sand barefoot. It was a cool and beautiful day in January, and I was rejoicing over His sweet presence. As I walked in the warmth of the sun on our beach, I came to a part where there are a million grey and black rocks. God drew me to a pretty red rock about an inch wide. I heard him say, "This is a reminder of the Word I gave you to slay your giant with." Because I heard his voice and walked in it, that giant was slain with one small stone. He was beheaded! It only took one!

Out of all those rocks, He had predestined only this one to lead me to victory! Walking along the shallow waves hearing his powerful whispers, He brought to mind the words that He spoke to me that carried me through to victory as I clenched that rock to my heart! These words of pure gold, my most precious possession, and nothing could ever take them away!

I can tell you with all surety that if I were to go through the past 20 years again, knowing what I know now, my outcome would have been so different every step of the way. God could have reached down and rescued me at any moment through all those years, but He didn't. He had to walk me through until I could see Him in the fire, until I could see how He loves me, and so that I could truly understand who He is. The fire is the only place where I could learn the greatness of my God. I had to learn some painful lessons for myself and for others.

Now, all the words, revelations, and wisdom He taught me in 2018 and 2019 are not just tucked away for a rainy day, but they are blooming. They are giving life and hope to others, armor for each battle in the future. God did not just prepare me for the present battle, but the future ones too.

You cannot win today's battle on yesterday's revelation. From glory to glory we must go! This is our path. Each victory planted many seeds of faith for the next fight, the new season. For these new seeds to grow, we must remain steadfast in the rain of His presence. With each battle coming, new strategies, greater strengths, and wisdom will arise. New battle plans will be given to me. Each victory will be sweeter than the last.

I was so amazed at God when He showed me that this victory reached farther than I ever imagined. When it was over, He spoke far more blessings over my life than the amount of suffering I had endured for all those years. Those battles that I thought were lost in the past were now being transformed into victories by Him, changing the effects of all those defeats by changing my heart, my understanding of them, and what they taught me. He was truly taking what the enemy meant for evil and turned it around for His glory, creating beauty out of them.

They no longer have power over me, except to show me where His mercy carried me through, and to show how evident God's love is for me. They cause me no more tears, but only shouts of joy because of my gratefulness to God. Those things that caused me so much fear, now cause me to laugh at the devil and proclaim victory for others. He taught me so much from what were once defeats, but now are my reasons to prevail.

Although this victory was incredible, He spoke to me about how this was only the beginning, the foundation for what He would reveal to me about the victories I would have in the future, and about the battles I would walk with Him through, and the fullness of my life I would walk in because of it.

One day, while I was recovering, I was overtaken in worship as He whispered to me His infinite love once again, "I have turned your bitter waters into wine." Nothing was lost in all those years of pain and suffering because God told me, *"Every tear was now the anointing oil that I will use to show those living in defeat how I can lead them to live victoriously."* This oil that He brought forth from the crushing of my soul for His purpose—expensive and perfumed, but now, finally, I could pray for others.

All the suffering and pain I had been through in 20 years—all the bloodshed, all the scars—could have never been enough to save me, to pay the price for my life. Jesus was the only one that could do that, but now all of it paved the way for me to understand God in order to bring this light to the lost. This was a price too high for many to pay, but worth every tear I see on their faces. When I say to someone on the streets, "God loves you," it comes out of me with fierceness and unstoppable love. When I give of myself to a person in need, I know it's out of a force of the love of God that is unstoppable, reaching out through me. When I reach out to pray for someone, joy fills my heart because I know the incredible love of the Father for them. The presence of God wants to pour out of me. His words want to reach out to their hearts!

Meditation Scriptures

1 Samuel 14:47 NLT

Now when Saul had secured his grasp on Israel's throne, he fought against his enemies in every direction—against Moab, Ammon, Edom, the kings of Zobah, and the Philistines. *And wherever he turned, he was victorious.*

Psalm 121:7-8 NKJV

The Lord shall preserve you from all evil;
He shall preserve your soul.
The Lord shall preserve your going out and your coming in
From this time forth, and even forevermore.

Song of Songs 8:6 (TPT)

Fasten me upon your heart as a seal of fire forevermore. This living, consuming flame will seal you as my prisoner of love. My passion is stronger than the chains of death and the grave, all consuming as the very flashes of fire from the burning heart of God. Place this fierce, unrelenting fire over your entire being.

Exodus 15:22-25 AMP

Then Moses led Israel from the Red Sea, and they went into the Wilderness of Shur; they went [a distance of] three days (about thirty-three miles) in the wilderness and found no water. Then they came to Marah, but they could not drink its waters because they were bitter; therefore it was named Marah (bitter).

The people [grew discontented and] grumbled at Moses, saying, "What are we going to drink?" Then he cried to the Lord [for help], and the Lord showed him a tree, [a branch of] which he threw into the waters, and the waters became sweet.

Isaiah 38:16-17 NLT

Lord, your discipline is good, for it leads to life and health. You restore my health
and allow me to live!
Yes, this anguish was good for me, for you have rescued me from death
and forgiven all my sins.

Psalm 103:2-5 MSG

O my soul, bless God.
From head to toe, I'll bless his holy name!
O my soul, bless God,
don't forget a single blessing!
He forgives your sins—every one.
He heals your diseases—every one.
He redeems you from hell—saves your life!
He crowns you with love and mercy—a paradise crown.
He wraps you in goodness—beauty eternal.
He renews your youth—you're always young in his presence.

Ephesians 4:31-32 NLT

Get rid of all bitterness, rage, anger, harsh words, and slander, as well as all types
of evil behavior. Instead, be kind to each other, tenderhearted, forgiving one
another, just as God through Christ has forgiven you.

CHAPTER 23: RESTORATION

"Above all, keep loving one another earnestly, since love covers a multitude of sins."

(1 Peter 4:8 ESV)

"But instead be kind and affectionate toward one another. Has God graciously forgiven you? Then graciously forgive one another in the depths of Christ's love."

(Ephesians 4:32 TPT)

God is faithful to every promise, no matter what it looks like in the natural! The things between me and my husband at some points were not only very disheartening and depressing, but very disturbing in the past 20 years. If not for God, I would have ended up in prison, and my husband would have been dead. I remember looking at him with such hate and rage at times that it scared me. Leaving or death was my only hope, and I wanted out so bad. That very little bit of desire for God, the mustard seed of hope He gave me at the beginning, was what He used to turn everything around. But I had to be obedient each step of the way, no matter how painful it was.

When I first started going to this church, I would sit down to have dinner with Elder Desirie about once a week and be filled with so much bitterness and pain telling her how I had to get out of this marriage. But by the time we left the restaurant, each time, a little more transformation had taken place in me. I would often joke that Mario was only alive right now because Elder Desirie saved his life. But in all reality, God had to save my life first!

A little more of my heart's broken pieces were put back together with each meal. Yes, I wanted Mario gone, but more so, I wanted God's will in my life. I wanted God's peace, and I wanted to surrender all of my life to God. And God wanted so much more for me and for us.

One day at a church picnic, we were there together, which was rare because we didn't do anything together, but yet so apart and God was stirring my heart. With tears in my eyes, I calmly said to Mario, "are we going to fix this mess or walk away." He said so confidently and with such authority, "God *will* fix this." I knew my husband was willing. But I just needed to let God show me the way. That is when much of the pain lifted, and I was able to let God into the ugliest part of my life.

Slowly, transformation in my behavior and thoughts changed as I let God take control, and slowly, our actions toward each other changed. I saw Mario in a different light, as God showed me how imperfect he was and how much he was in pain, much like me, but more so, that over the years his heart for God never changed. He had suffered, he had disappointments, he had frustrations, but he wanted God above all else.

Many times, it was like God was building a bridge piece by piece between us. As I took a step forward in obedience, another piece would fall into place. I could not see beyond that step I was taking right then, but trusted God with each new place we came to. I soon discovered that this bridge was much stronger than our original foundation.

When we came together to talk about God, I was amazed over and over again at the deep wells of wisdom and revelation within my husband that I never saw before. Many times, I would just eat of all the abundant fruit of revelation my husband had to share with me and kick myself for not knowing this sooner. It would frustrate me at times because my brain could not comprehend things he said which were so profound, but soon when I allowed God to speak to my heart through my husband, I saw the love he had for me behind it, and that's when my spirit began to understand and cry out for more.

One time, when we had a beautiful conversation pertaining to questions I had in a situation, I felt as though Mario was pouring the love of God on me like warm oil. When he left the room, I sat there in tears overwhelmed as my spirit was saturated with the greatness of God.

God took my marriage from tears of pain and rage, to tears of joy and peace. From brokenness, to wholeness within myself and my marriage. As well as forgiveness that washed away all that bitterness one tear at a time. It was not easy, but so, so, worth it. It's not yet perfect (mostly my fault), but we are willing and obedient.

CHAPTER 24:
SEASON OF PLUNDER

"This is what the Lord says: I will give Jerusalem a river of peace and prosperity. The wealth of the nations will flow to her."

(Isaiah 66:12a NLT)

"Yes, God is more than ready to overwhelm you with every form of grace, so that you will have more than enough of everything—every moment and in every way. He will make you overflow with abundance in every good thing you do."

(2 Corinthians 9:8 TPT)

I stood on the shores of His love, longing for Him, but I didn't know how to get into the depth of His love. For so long, I was on the outside looking in. I watched as the waves crashed over everyone else but me. But now I am submerged in Him, in His peace. He had overtaken me. He consumed me. That was all I wanted: His presence, His peace. I will not stand on the shore any longer. I will not hesitate at the sound of His voice. I will not fear. I will walk straight in every time, leaving behind everything on the shore that is not of God. Wave after wave of His love and blessing consumed my life. Wave after wave, He covers me in His grace and His mercy. Relentless waves of His presence always reviving, always refreshing, always soothing, and always peaceful, yet always fierce and powerful.

Right after the last surgery, God showed me a valley of rolling hills, and it was beautiful, lush, and green as far as the eye could see. It was very similar to a place I had seen when I was in Jerusalem, somewhere near the Sea of Galilee. He spoke to me that I was no longer in that dark valley I had been in for so long, but now I was walking into the valley of blessings. *I was now in the season that comes after the battle and victory, where joy is overflowing. A season of thankfulness. A time to gather the plunder, and a time of deep rest and rapid restoration. It was a season of walking in all of the promises!*

This was a time that cannot be explained with words! There was no stopping my worship! I wanted to leave my body so many times because I felt so limited in praising God! It was a time of continuous jubilee, peace like a river, strength like an army, a time of being saturated by God's presence, and blessing upon blessing. Over and over again, He has blessed me, and not only me, but those in my family and those close to me—all things I had never prayed for. Job promotions, new houses, new cars, and many wonderful blessings came to my children and grandchildren! The blessing of more of Him is my most precious treasure. Hearing God, seeing Him, knowing Him, is all I could ask for and all that satisfies me.

Many of the blessings He brought to me during this "season of plunder" were way above anything I could ask or think! In fact, I never asked for any of it. He just blessed me over and over again. It was a time where I just could not stop praising and worshiping God, and He ravished me daily with His sweet powerful presence. He was rejoicing with me!!!

During this time, *huge* amounts of money would come unexpectedly over and over again. I would receive so much favor everywhere I went. Everything I set my hands to do prospered beyond belief. God's grace overtook my life, and nothing was a struggle.

Then the most amazing miracle happened that I still cannot comprehend! God brought to me a grandson I never knew I had. DNA! Through my daughter donating her eggs years ago for couples to conceive that were unable to, a young couple out of New York had a baby boy. Sweet and silly 5-year-old Daniel who I fell in love with instantly! This beautiful boy's parents wanted me and my husband to be a part of his life! They wanted him to know all of his heritage.

I was so blown away because it was as though God was restoring to me that joy I had lost when I had lost my baby boy, Isaiah, many years back. He is always working behind the scenes on our behalf. This beautiful blessing had already been manifested 5 years ago, before I even knew about him! I had had a feeling like something was missing in my life for the past few years, and when they first contacted me, I knew God had completed that void in my life!

Another huge blessing during this season that we received was so overwhelming because of the fierce battle that we had helped my son through. We almost lost our granddaughter because of a bitter custody case we endured for so long. It was so heartbreaking watching our baby girl,

Addie, being fought over and used as a weapon against her father, all because of one person.

One day, out of the blue, God did a magnificent miracle, a truce was called by the most vicious and deceitful person in this battle, Addie's stepfather, Michael. He repented for his actions, and forgiveness was given on both sides; there would be no more fighting and there would only be unity. As a result, my son's child support was willingly reduced drastically, and he received much more visitation! But God went even further, and they reconciled so much of the pain of the past, that they became friends, watching each other's kids and attending birthday parties and recitals together.

Without being asked, my son found it in his heart to allow Addie's new stepdad's last name to be added to my granddaughter's name legally, bringing much more restoration to everyone. I was so, so, proud of him! Now she is so excited to be Adelynn Grace Soto-McAllister. She knows that she does not have two families anymore. She has one big happy family in two houses, and everyone loves everyone! My God is AMAZING!

God was doing so much in me after I came home from the hospital. Some of these beautiful blessings He did were not *for* me, but *through* me—which was even better, and was a part of this incredible season of plunder! A season that is not just for you, but for those around you. So much plunder that you can bless so many others. God did something amazing through my giving. nIt was not about just helping others anymore, but an act of pure love that could not be contained.

I had been a craft supply hoarder for years, and had 6 large crates of yarn, and God impressed on my heart to start making hats and scarves as I was recovering. So that is what I did. Our winters are very cold, but it's the strong wind that makes it unbearable. The scarves and hats were super thick, warm, and soft, and as soon as I had 10 sets made, I started to hand them out to the homeless in our area. Altogether, over 3 months, I handed out about 100 sets. They absolutely loved them, and with that, they received the Word of God and books and blankets.

One day, as I was driving home, and on a street corner sitting in the cold, there was a very thin young man with an empty cart and thin jacket. He had his head in his hands as though he were very sad or crying. I immediately pulled over and asked him if he was ok, and if he wanted a hat and scarf. He said, "yes, please," and started to cry. He said he had nothing left, I could see all he had was the clothes on his back and his cart. So, with the scarf set, I gave him pillows, a large down comforter, some food, and the Word of God! This was so wonderful and life changing for both of us. I knew this was the critical moment in his life and that only God could have destined for us to meet to show him he was deeply loved.

Soon after that is when the world pandemic of 2020 hit. I had no idea what God was going to do next, but I decided my "yes" would not be intermittent or just when it is convenient. So, as God leads, I follow. This is why it is so important to be led by the spirit of God in everything. I sewed a mask for my granddaughter, and everyone loved it! The timing was perfect. God once again used my craft stockpile of 5 huge boxes of fabric to make hundreds and hundreds of masks for people with virus filters inside of them.

He just showed me exactly what to do. And my family joined in and helped. We had so many orders we could not keep up. We worked tirelessly for 10-14 hours a day for several months cutting and sewing. The grace of God carried us through like never before! Because of this, we were able to feed many families that were not working from the proceeds.

I could have never imagined such a blessing happening, but this season of plunder was incredible! The Valley of Blessing is a place of such incredible spiritual wealth that you cannot contain it all!

Meditation Scriptures

Psalm 84:5-7 TPT

How enriched are they who find their strength in the Lord;
within their hearts are the highways of holiness!
Even when their paths wind through the dark valley of tears,
they dig deep to find a pleasant pool *where others find only pain.*
He gives to them a brook of blessing
filled from the rain of an outpouring.
They grow stronger and stronger with every step forward,
and the God of all gods will appear before them in Zion.

Psalms 126:5-6 TPT

Those who sow their tears as seeds will reap a harvest with joyful shouts of glee. They may weep as they go out carrying their seed to sow, but they will return with joyful laughter and shouting with gladness as they bring back armloads of blessing and a harvest overflowing!

Isaiah 65:24 BSB

Even before they call, I will answer, and while they are still speaking, I will hear.

Psalm 40:3 AMP

He put a new song in my mouth, a song of praise to our God;
Many will see and fear [with great reverence]
And will trust confidently in the Lord.

2 Chronicles 20:20-27 NLT

Early the next morning the army of Judah went out into the wilderness of Tekoa. On the way Jehoshaphat stopped and said, "Listen to me, all you people of Judah and Jerusalem! Believe in the Lord your God, and you will be able to stand firm. Believe in his prophets, and you will succeed."

After consulting the people, the king appointed singers to walk ahead of the army, singing to the Lord and praising him for his holy splendor. This is what they sang:

"Give thanks to the Lord; his faithful love endures forever!"

At the very moment they began to sing and give praise, the Lord caused the armies of Ammon, Moab, and Mount Seir to start fighting among themselves. The armies of Moab and Ammon turned against their allies from Mount Seir and killed every one of them. After they had destroyed the army of Seir, they began attacking each other.

So when the army of Judah arrived at the lookout point in the wilderness, all they saw were dead bodies lying on the ground as far as they could see. Not a single one of the enemy had escaped.

King Jehoshaphat and his men went out to gather the plunder. They found vast amounts of equipment, clothing, and other valuables—more than they could carry. There was so much plunder that it took them three days just to collect it all! On the fourth day they gathered in the Valley of Blessing, which got its name that day because the people praised and thanked the Lord there. It is still called the Valley of Blessing today.

Then all the men returned to Jerusalem, with Jehoshaphat leading them, overjoyed that *the Lord had given them victory over their enemies.*

Galatians 5:25 NLT

Since we are living by the Spirit, let us follow the Spirit's leading in every part of our lives.

1 Peter 1:6-7 NLT

So be truly glad. *There is wonderful joy ahead,* even though you must endure many trials for a little while. These trials will show that your faith is genuine. It is being tested as fire tests and purifies gold—though your faith is far more precious than mere gold. So when your faith remains strong through many trials, it will bring you much praise and glory and honor on the day when Jesus Christ is revealed to the whole world.

Isaiah 1:19 TPT

If you have a willing heart to let me help you,
and if you will obey me, you will feast on the blessings
of an abundant harvest.

Numbers 6:24-26 AMP

The Lord bless you, and keep you [protect you, sustain you, and guard you];
The Lord make His face shine upon you [with favor],
And be gracious to you [surrounding you with lovingkindness];
The Lord lift up His countenance (face) upon you [with divine approval],
And give you peace [a tranquil heart and life].

EPILOGUE

"So why would I fear the future? For your goodness and love pursue me all the days of my life. Then afterward, when my life is through, I'll return to your glorious presence to be forever with you!"
(Psalms 23:6 TPT)

"*Adonai*'s right hand is lifted high! *Adonai*'s right hand is mighty!" I will not die, but live, and proclaim what *Adonai* has done!"

(Psalms 118:16-17 TLV)

When they first told me I had cancer, I never expected to live this long—but God! The devil made me believe I had an expiration date because my mom died 10 years after her first diagnosis—but God! It's now been 12 years to the day since I was first diagnosed! Now, I am stronger, wiser, and fearless. I do not let anything stand in my way of living. Now, my life is so different. At 58, whatever God allows me to do, I enjoy it to the fullest. No fear, no hesitation! Whether it be ministry in other countries or enjoying my grandkids. Every chance I get, I am traveling all over the world, taking long road trips, hiking with my family, going on photography trips, camping, taking firearm classes, going to every beach I can, taking exercise classes, paddle boarding, snorkeling, etc. There is so much more I want to do! I walked through a very dark valley for so long, but now I am living in the Valley of Blessings!

Isaiah 61:3 ESV

To grant to those who mourn in Zion— to give them a beautiful headdress instead of ashes, the oil of gladness instead of mourning, the garment of praise instead of a faint spirit; that they may be called oaks of righteousness, the planting of the Lord, that he may be glorified.

Ecclesiastes 3:11 NLT

Yet God has made everything beautiful for its own time. He has planted eternity in the human heart, but even so, people cannot see the whole scope of God's work from beginning to end.

One of the main things God wanted to show me during this time of plunder was His deep love for me and how I am to love. He loved me when I couldn't love or look at myself in the mirror. He loved me through every tear, He loved me through every heartache. He loved me despite my rebellion, my bitterness, my ugliness. It no longer mattered what others said or did, I was loved so deeply by almighty God that nothing else mattered.

He taught me the meaning of true beauty. What you may see with your eyes is not the meaning of beauty at all. Real beauty cannot be seen. You will never hear me say to someone that they are beautiful for their physical traits because that is not what I see. We must look beyond the mirror, beyond the photos, beyond the superficial.

EPILOGUE

Beauty is who God is in us. I could not be the world's definition of beautiful which was so temporary and futile. So, I determined in my heart I would be God's definition of beautiful, even if nobody else could see it, I knew my Father could see it. That is where the real satisfaction comes from. Receiving praise for your physical beauty is fruitless and only promotes vanity, which is nothing compared to when God says that you belong to Him, that you are His beautiful treasure, and that He is pleased with you. These words are what I craved, what I sought after.

As I was standing in the bathroom after a shower one day, Gods' presence surprised me once again. He drew my attention to my scars, now 23, and as I looked at them, I began to weep just like the last time. But this time, it was different. It was cleansing, refreshing, and as though it was a peaceful pain. I felt so many emotions from all the years of shame, bitterness, loneliness, and pain, that suddenly all reappeared.

I had thought I was healed from all this, and I was, but God had to show me one last thing. They no longer had any effect on me. As I ran my hand over the many scars, suddenly, my wedding ring's diamonds began to glisten so brightly like never before, as God spoke so gently to my spirit, "This is how I see you." Never was I so overtaken before! There could be no greater love!

I now look at my disfigured body and aging face, and say, "I trust you God because I am your beloved." I now feel symptoms in my body and say, "I trust you God because I AM blessed." I get devastating news and I say, "I trust you God because I KNOW you are faithful." Not mere words, but actions and power coming straight from my spirit because I AM BLESSED.

My scars are now evidence of His deep faithful love for me, His salvation over my life, His healing power that was paid for by the blood of Jesus. One day after the last surgery, I was sitting at my desk overwhelmed by His presence while I quietly worshipped Him as He gently and powerfully proclaimed over me, **"You are branded by my love!"** No Longer branded by fear, pain, and torment, but by the scars Jesus endured for me. I am branded as Jesus was by the love of God for us! Every scar, every tear, every prayer, and every broken piece of my heart, now had meaning, and now I know nothing was ever in vain. His goodness is evident in every stitch that holds me together! These ashes were being transformed into the beauty He always intended me to walk in!

This battle wasn't about me. It was about Him all along and who HE is to me and in me. "Who do you say that I AM". I say you are wonderful, you are faithful, you are the lover of my soul, you are all I desire, you are everything to me Lord!

EPILOGUE

Meditation Scriptures

1 Corinthians 13:1-8a TPT

If I were to speak with eloquence in earth's many languages, and in the heavenly tongues of angels, yet I didn't express myself with love, my words would be reduced to the hollow sound of nothing more than a clanging cymbal.
And if I were to have the gift of prophecy with a profound understanding of God's hidden secrets, and if I possessed unending supernatural knowledge, and if I had the greatest gift of faith that could move mountains, but have never learned to love, then I am nothing.
And if I were to be so generous as to give away everything I owned to feed the poor, and to offer my body to be burned as a martyr, without the pure motive of love,

I would gain nothing of value.

Love is large and incredibly patient. Love is gentle and consistently kind to all. It refuses to be jealous when blessing comes to someone else. Love does not brag about one's achievements nor inflate its own importance. Love does not traffic in shame and disrespect, nor selfishly seek its own honor. Love is not easily irritated or quick to take offense. Love joyfully celebrates honesty and finds no delight in what is wrong. Love is a safe place of shelter, for it never stops believing the best for others. Love never takes failure as defeat, for it never gives up. Love never stops loving.

Proverbs 3:3-4 AMP

Do not let mercy and kindness and truth leave you [instead let these qualities define you]; Bind them [securely] around your neck, Write them on the tablet of your heart. So find favor and high esteem In the sight of God and man.

Isaiah 61:7 BSB

Instead of shame, My people will have a double portion, and instead of humiliation, they will rejoice in their share; and so they will inherit a double portion in their land, and everlasting joy will be theirs.

Isaiah 61:1-3 ESV

The Spirit of the Lord God is upon me, because the Lord has anointed me to bring good news to the poor; he has sent me to bind up the brokenhearted, to proclaim liberty to the captives, and the opening of the prison to those who are bound; to proclaim the year of the Lord's favor, and the day of vengeance of our God; to comfort all who mourn; to grant to those who mourn in Zion—to give them a beautiful headdress instead of ashes, the oil of gladness instead of mourning, the garment of praise instead of a faint spirit; that they may be called oaks of righteousness, the planting of the Lord, that he may be glorified.

Isaiah 66:2 BSB

Has not My hand made all these things? And so they came into being," declares the LORD. "This is the one I will esteem: he who is humble and contrite in spirit, who trembles at My word.

Exodus 13:8-9 NLT

"On the seventh day you must explain to your children, 'I am celebrating what the Lord did for me when I left Egypt.' This annual festival will be a visible sign to you, like a mark branded on your hand or your forehead. Let it remind you always to recite this teaching of the Lord: 'With a strong hand, the Lord rescued you from Egypt.'"

EPILOGUE

Ephesians 1:13-14 NIV

And you also were included in Christ when you heard the message of truth, the gospel of your salvation. When you believed, you were marked in him with a seal, the promised Holy Spirit, who is a deposit guaranteeing our inheritance until the redemption of those who are God's possession—to the praise of his glory.

1 Corinthians 1:21-22 BSB

Now it is God who establishes both us and you in Christ. He anointed us, placed His seal on us, and put His Spirit in our hearts as a pledge of what is to come.

Galatians 6:17 NLT

From now on, don't let anyone trouble me with these things. For I bear on my body the scars that show I belong to Jesus.

Ephesians 4:30 AMP

And do not grieve the Holy Spirit of God [but seek to please Him], by whom you were sealed *and* marked [branded as God's own] for the day of redemption [the final deliverance from the consequences of sin].

Isaiah 43:13

"Even from eternity I am He, And there is none who can deliver out of My hand; I act and who can reverse it?"

Psalms 143:11 NLT

For the glory of your name, O Lord, preserve my life. Because of your faithfulness, bring me out of this distress.

Psalms 31:19 TPT

Lord, how wonderful you are! You have stored up so many good things for us, like a treasure chest heaped up and spilling over with blessings—all for those who honor and worship you! Everybody knows what you can do for those who turn and hide themselves in you.

Luke 1:45 TPT

Great favor is upon you, for you have believed every word spoken to you from the Lord."

Psalms 32:8-9 TPT

I hear the Lord saying, "I will stay close to you, instructing and guiding you along the pathway for your life.

I will advise you along the way and lead you forth with my eyes as your guide.

So don't make it difficult; don't be stubborn when I take you where you've not been before. Don't make me tug you and pull you along. Just come with me!"

ACKNOWLEDGMENT

First and foremost I want to thank my husband Mario, for his faithfulness to God. He was always my lighthouse during this long relentless storm even when I didn't realize it and even when I gave him every reason to leave. That glimmer of light was always something I looked for in the darkness. I look back at all the years and things we went through and during that time his love for God never changed. Because of his relationship with God and the abundance of beautiful revelation he has shared with me, Mario has helped to pull me out of my darkest days. Despite all the devastation, the battles, through all the misery, he still loves me. For his tenacity to stay together and stay by my side, I will be forever indebted and grateful.

When God brought my fierce friend, Desirie Canedos into my life, he knew exactly what I needed that no one else had. There is no greater love than to lay down your life for a friend unconditionally and never asking anything in return and she did this with her whole heart. It was not easy to be around her and hear her truthful words at times, but I was like a person that was so thirsty for the truth. There could be no compromising, no sugar coating, and no backing down and that is exactly how she approached everything with me with a love and compassion that far surpasses what I thought possible. God did more through her, then I could do on my own. For her unselfish heart, I will be forever beholden and appreciative.

ABOUT THE AUTHOR

Patricia Soto is a wife, mother of 4, grandmother of 7, photographer, and philanthropist. Prior to retiring from the San Bernardino County Sheriff's Department, she worked supervising inmate work crews.

One of Patrcia's greatest passions is to see those with cancer healed and walk in victory. To fulfill this passion, Patricia volunteers for a hospital's program called "No One Dies Alone." Through this program she, along with others, are given the opportunity to sit with and minister to those that are in their last hours.

When Patricia isn't volunteering at the hospital, she is busy serving in her local church. Over the years she has served as a leader, hospitality assistant, assistant to a pastor, as well as a shut-in services coordinator. For the last 5 years Patricia has also been afforded the opportunity to use her 10 years of experience as a photographer to capture thousands of hours for many church events located in the United States as well as Brazil and Mexico.

Her heart of servitude extends far beyond her local church. Patricia loves giving to the homeless, orphanages in Brazil and Mexico, and anywhere there is a need. Infact, she has been involved in helping to take thousands of dollars worth of clothing and food to Brazil ministries.

Patricia currently resides in California with her family.

www.ingramcontent.com/pod-product-compliance
Lightning Source LLC
Chambersburg PA
CBHW051040160426
43193CB00010B/1019